The Hilton Head Over-35 Diet

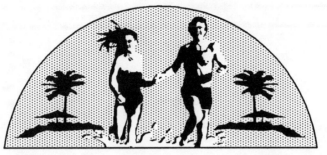

T H E
Hilton Head
Over–35
D I E T

**Change Your Metabolism:
Look and Feel
Years Younger**

Dr. Peter M. Miller

WARNER BOOKS

A Warner Communications Company

This book is *not* intended as a substitute for the medical advice of physicians. The reader should regularly consult a physician in matters relating to his or her health and particularly in respect to any symptoms that may require diagnosis or medical treatment.

Warner Books, Inc., 666 Fifth Avenue, New York, NY 10103

W A Warner Communications Company

Printed in the United States of America

First printing: January 1989

10 9 8 7 6 5 4 3 2 1

Library of Congress Cataloging-in-Publication Data

Miller, Peter M. (Peter Michael), 1942–
The Hilton Head over-35 diet: change your metabolism: look and feel years younger / Peter M. Miller.
    p.   cm.
Produced in cooperation with the staff of the Hilton Head Health Institute.
    Bibliography: p. 207
    Includes index.
    1. Middle age—Health and hygiene.   2. Middle age—Nutrition.
3. Reducing diets.   4. Exercise.   I. Hilton Head Health Institute.
II. Title.
RA777.5.M55 1989
613'.0434—dc19   88-18869
ISBN 0-446-51430-6   CIP

Illustrations by Peter Michael Miller, Jr.

Book design by H. Roberts

*This book is dedicated to
"Dr." Don Christy, whose timely professional
assistance has been invaluable to my career*

ACKNOWLEDGMENTS

The program described in this book represents the product of years of effort and input from my staff at the Hilton Head Health Institute. I am greatly indebted to them for their continuing contributions to the content and development of the Hilton Head Over-35 Diet. I would especially like to acknowledge the assistance of Robert Wright, Dr. Howard Rankin, Tom Miller, Hunter Smith, Dr. Roger Sargent, and my wife, Gabrielle.

I am particularly grateful to all of the over-35 men and women who have participated in our programs at the Hilton Head Health Institute and who have so graciously shared their lives with us.

CONTENTS

Contents

Contents

Introduction

Jane is a 39-year-old career woman, wife, and mother whose weight problems may be very similar to yours. In her early 20s Jane weighed 120 pounds, a good, healthy weight for her 5-foot, 5-inch frame. She took pride in her trim figure and was always attractively dressed. While she occasionally had a problem with an extra five or six pounds, with a little dieting she was usually back to her normal weight in about a week.

Now, at age 39, her life has changed and so has her weight. Jane owns and manages a small but elite women's clothing shop and along with her husband Alex, a district sales manager for a computer company, raises two sons, Jeffery, age 12 and Robert, age 9.

Starting about five years ago Jane found that she was having more and more of a difficult time maintaining her 120-pound weight. Admittedly, she wasn't as physically active as she once was, but she still played tennis every weekend and went for bike rides with Alex a couple of evenings a week. In spite of her best efforts, her scale now usually registered between 128 and 132. What was especially frustrating to her was the fact that she did not seem to be eating much more than she did ten years ago.

Dieting frustrated Jane even more. No longer could she follow a low-calorie diet and lose five to six pounds in a week. Rather, she had to struggle to lose even two pounds a week. Jane put it this way:

> **Last week I went on the same diet I used to follow when I was 20. It worked great for me then, but now my body just won't respond in the same way. I didn't realize that age could slow my body down so much. Even when I lose weight after several weeks of dieting, I put it all right back on before I know it.**

Jane began to worry a great deal about her weight. She went from one fad diet to another only to experience temporary results. Her weight affected her self-image. She began to think of herself as "frumpy" and, worse yet, "matronly." Then, even Alex began to tease her about her weight. She realized, however, that her excess poundage was no laughing matter and if she didn't do something about the problem, her self-respect, peace of mind, and even her marriage would suffer.

Don is a 44-year-old tax attorney who is married to Jeanne, a 41-year-old artist. While Jeanne has been able to maintain her youthful figure, Don had developed a substantial weight problem over the past ten years. At his latest medical exam, he weighed in at 220 pounds, much too heavy for his six-foot height. Because of his large, athletic frame he always looked good in college with a weight of 180 pounds. But, at 220, he definitely looked fat and out of shape. And he had more to worry about. His doctor discovered that he had a high cholesterol level and that his blood-sugar level was high enough to put him into a prediabetic category.

Don knew he had to lose his weight and lose it for good. Past diets worked for a short time but the weight always came back in a few weeks. What confused him most was the fact that, although he'd always had a hearty appetite, he could always get away with it (at least for the first 35 years of his life) as far as his weight was concerned.

These were Don's words of frustration and worry when he first consulted me about his dilemma:

> Doctor Miller, I used to be able to control my weight fairly well. Oh, I might put on a few pounds during the winter months or on a vacation trip but I could get them off just by exercising a little more. As I got older, things changed. Now, over the past few years I've put on 40 pounds. I don't eat any more than I did when I was younger. My body just isn't burning calories like it once did. If I don't do something to spark up my metabolism now, I'll weigh over 250 pounds by the time I'm 50. You've got to help me!

If these cases remind you of your own efforts to lose weight after the age of 35, believe me, you're not alone. If you've never experienced a problem with your weight before age 35, you surely will now. If you had a weight problem while you were young, it is likely to worsen after 35.

In fact:

MOST PEOPLE GAIN 15 TO 25 POUNDS BETWEEN THE AGES OF 35 AND 55

Before I run the risk of depressing you about your weight difficulties, let me assure you that I understand your problem completely. And, more importantly, I believe I have the solution to your over-35 fat problem.

Why I Can Cure Your Over-35 Weight Problem

Twelve years ago, after nearly 13 years of experience in the research field, I established the Hilton Head Health Institute, an in-residence health clinic on Hilton Head Island, South Carolina. As a clinical psychologist specializing in health habits, I had long been concerned with the lack of cooperation among professionals dealing with obesity. In spite of the fact that almost everyone admits that weight control is a complex, multidimensional problem, diet books and diet programs continue to approach overweight from one particular bias or another. For example, one program might emphasize a strictly medical solution to the problem, another might stress nutrition education, still another might say the answer lies totally in behavior modification. My aim was to bring together the expertise of clinicians and researchers with different professional backgrounds to examine every single aspect of the weight-control issue from metabolism to motivation.

My dream was to create a top-of-the-line clinical and research facility staffed by experts in the fields of nutrition, medicine, exercise physiology, and behavioral psychology who could come up with scientific, no-nonsense answers to the problem of overweight.

Now, a dozen years after its inception, the Hilton Head Health Institute enjoys an international reputation for being one of the top professional programs in the field of weight control. Thousands of men and women from all over the United States as well as other countries such as Great Britain, Canada, Switzerland, France, and Italy have completed our treatment program and are now living slim, fat-free lives.

The Institute has provided my colleagues and myself a unique opportunity to study weight problems very intensively on a day-to-day basis. This research has been going on for almost 13 years and was first outlined in my best-selling book, *The Hilton Head Metabolism Diet*.

Beyond the Hilton Head Metabolism Diet

In spite of the fact that the Hilton Head Metabolism Diet is so successful, we have continued to look for ways to improve upon our past discoveries. In addition, I have become more and more concerned about the plight of the over-35 age group in their struggles with weight control. This interest was spurred by the fact that we were seeing more and more over-35 people at the Institute and were observing, firsthand, the metabolic slowdown they were experiencing. In addition, since I am 45 years of age I can relate in a very direct and personal way to this problem. I am not overweight, simply because I practice what I preach, but I would be if I did not actively stir up my metabolism by using the Hilton Head Over-35 Diet plan.

I have found that over-35 men and women need a special dietary program because they must ward off the damaging effects of age on the body's natural fat-burning system.

The Promise of Eternal Youth?

No. Unfortunately, I cannot offer you the promise of eternal youth. However, using the Hilton Head Over-35 Diet you can recondition your body, revitalize your metabolism, and make yourself feel the way you did years ago.

I've heard so many of my clients tell me that they feel young again. One of them put it this way:

Your Hilton Head Over-35 Diet has worked miracles for me. I look younger and, more importantly, I feel younger. Since

I lost 30 pounds my friends say I look 38 instead of 48! I used to be so sluggish and now I'm full of energy and vitality. I walk for an hour every day and have never felt better. Now I realize that just because I'm getting older I don't have to be fat. I don't have to be tired all the time. I finally feel in control of my body and I'm looking forward to being slim for the rest of my life.

Your New Lease on Life

Now that you are over 35 years of age you must remember that ordinary diets will no longer work for you. Overeating is not your major problem. You are overweight because the aging process has suppressed your body's normal ability to burn calories through metabolism. Because of this fact the solution to your weight problem is not simply giving up eating for the rest of your life.

What you need is a program designed not only to help you lose weight but also to change your body chemistry to give you a younger metabolism. What most people (and even some doctors) don't realize is that metabolic activity can be controlled. It can be increased by as much as 500 calories a day. That means that, at rest, while you are standing, sitting, or even sleeping, your body will have shifted into higher gear, burning calories as if it were younger. I've seen it happen for thousands of others and I know it can happen for you.

My Hilton Head Over-35 Diet will provide you with:

- A diet that will turn your sluggish metabolism into a younger, more vital one
- Special age-related nutrition that your over-35 body requires for energy, stamina, and fitness
- Four satisfying meals each day during the week

- Five meals and more calories on the weekends to allow you more flexibility for entertaining and eating out
- Foods that are easy to prepare and even easier to obtain in restaurants or while traveling
- A low-impact exercise program designed to avoid injuries and fit into your busy schedule
- Specially designed exercises to enable you to develop a firm, trim, younger-looking body
- A mental reconditioning program designed to provide a younger frame of mind to go along with your younger body

Your Personal Diet Consultation

As you read *The Hilton Head Over-35 Diet* keep in mind that this is much more than a diet book. I want you to think of it as a personal consultation with me and the members of my staff. You are being advised by experts in nutrition, medicine, biology, behavioral psychology, and exercise physiology. You are also benefiting from the experience we've had in helping thousands of people just like you at the Hilton Head Health Institute.

In fact, I'd like you to imagine that, through this book, you are enrolling in the Institute. Now get ready to revitalize your metabolism. You and I are going to supercharge your fat-burning engine and rediscover the firm, slim body of your youth!

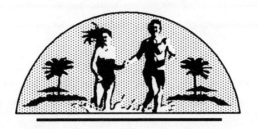

Age-Related Weight Problems

While there certainly are those few people who age gracefully, eating anything and everything and not gaining an ounce, they are an exception to the rule. Fortunately for them they were born with an extremely high metabolism and are able to get away with eating whatever they want in spite of the bodily changes that take place with age. Don't you just hate them!

I have a friend who is in this category. He has been thin all of his life. At 42 years of age he is 6-foot-1 and weighs a total of 142 pounds. His weight hasn't changed one ounce in the past 20 years in spite of the fact that he eats like a glutton and never, ever exercises. He even gave up smoking last year with no associated weight gain.

Rather than be happy with his lot in life, my friend complains about his size, looking for ways to put on weight. A few months ago he had the "brilliant" idea of wanting to come to my Institute to give a talk on the personal trauma of being chronically thin. When I told a group of my clients about his suggestion, the response was unanimous—laughter followed by tongue-in-cheek threats to lynch him if he ever came near the place!

Obviously, my friend is an exception to the rule. Most people, like yourself, gain weight as the years go on. With what we know about the aging process and how it affects metabolism, weight gain with age is practically inevitable.

The Facts and Figures

Let me share some statistics with you to drive this point home. The following chart shows very clearly how weight problems increase with age. For each age category the numbers indicate the percentage of men and women who are 10 percent or more above their ideal weights.

PERCENT OF UNITED STATES POPULATION IN VARYING AGE GROUPS WHO ARE OVERWEIGHT

Age	Women	Men
20–29	23%	31%
30–39	41%	53%
40–49	59%	60%
50–59	67%	63%
60–69	68%	57%

These figures are startling. Notice the marked increase in the prevalence of weight problems as people age. What is astonishing and what truly illustrates the major point of *The Hilton Head Over-35 Diet* is that the percentage of men and women who are overweight practically doubles from the mid-20s to the mid to late 30s.

Another impressive fact is related to the sheer number of over-35 adults who are overweight. By age 50 about two-thirds of the population of the United States weigh more than is healthy for them!

You'll also notice that, for men, prevalence of weight problems decreases after the 50–59 age category. Most experts feel that this is related to what is called the "survivor phenomenon." That is, percentages are no longer increasing simply because more of the overweight group is dying off and no longer included in the statistical sample. I'm sure that makes you feel a little uneasy. I know it does me. This is one type of study in which I wouldn't want to be considered a "dropout."

How Do We Compare with Other Countries?

Research conducted in other countries supports these conclusions and demonstrates that age-related weight problems are universal. This is not surprising since we all have the same physiology and our metabolisms deteriorate the same way whether we are British, Italian, or Chinese.

It is interesting to note, however, that, compared to Canada and Great Britain, the United States has a greater prevalence of weight problems especially in the upper age categories. Young women in our country (between the ages of 20 and 24) are actually in better physical shape than their British or Canadian counterparts. With age, however, these differences disappear, with American women in the 45–54 age group far surpassing both countries in percentage of the population who are overweight. American men are more overweight than men in the other countries in all age categories.

These cultural differences seem to be due to the fact that

the British and Canadians remain more physically active throughout their lives. Physical activity is incorporated into their life-styles to a greater extent than is true in our country. For example, the British are less dependent on automobile transportation and are more likely to walk to shops, neighbors' homes, or even to the railroad station to commute to work. Physical activity in the United States is much more centered around structured exercise routines or athletics, both of which tend to diminish with age.

Is Age-Related Overweight Inevitable?

Your body will certainly try to make you fatter as you get older, but you don't have to put up with it. If you do nothing to fight the effects of age on your metabolism, I can guarantee you will gradually gain weight each year for the rest of your life.

Many people who consult me have the mistaken impression that as they age they are supposed to be fat. One woman said:

> **But, doctor, I'm 53 years old. I couldn't possibly weigh what I did when I was 25. I believe I'm at the right weight for my age.**

These comments were made with serious intent in spite of the fact that this woman was 35 pounds over her ideal, healthy weight!

Remember: Getting older is no excuse for getting fatter.

There is no reason why you can't weigh the same at 60 as you did when you were 20. Saying it's not possible or not healthy is a cop-out. It's an excuse that's dangerous because it shows you are becoming complacent with yourself, your appearance, and, perhaps, even your life.

It is easy to fall into this frame of mind. It is easy to get discouraged. If this has happened to you, let's put all that in the past. I want to give you a new body, a more youthful appearance, and a new life.

Why Getting Fatter Will Make You Older

In this chapter I showed you the figures that indicate that getting older will make you fatter. Well, the reverse is also true. Getting fatter will make you look and feel older, perhaps as much as ten years older.

I'm sure you are fully aware of the toll that being overweight takes on your medical health, particularly after the age of 35. High blood pressure is 5.6 times more likely if you are overweight than if you are not. You are also more prone to cholesterol problems and diabetes. Overweight men are more likely to develop cancer of the colon and prostate while overweight women are more susceptible to cancer of the breast and uterus.

The good news is that once you lose your excess weight these health-risk factors disappear. At the Hilton Head Health Institute we regularly see significant reductions in blood pressure, blood cholesterol levels, and blood-sugar levels as our clients lose weight. And most of these improvements occur in as little as four weeks!

For men, there is even evidence to suggest that older-age impotence is caused by the same cardiovascular-disease risk factors associated with overweight. Losing weight and eating properly may, indeed, have the added benefit of improving your sex life!

While health issues frequently serve to motivate someone to go on a diet, they seldom help with the long-term commitment required to continue following a healthy life-style plan. The effect is very short-lived.

Are You a Candidate for the Over-35 Diet?

Check off each of the following characteristics that applies to you:

1. I am between 35 and 75 years of age.
2. I put on weight more easily now than when I was younger.
3. As the years progress my body is flabbier and not as firm as it once was.
4. I am not as physically active as I was during my youth.
5. I don't lose weight as quickly on diets as I once did.
6. Even when I lose weight on diets, I seem to gain it back more quickly than used to be the case.
7. I have more trouble being consistent with dieting and exercise than I once did.
8. I have a more difficult time motivating myself to start a diet than I did when I was younger (I keep putting it off).
9. I feel older than I should for my age.
10. My body is not as energetic as it once was.

The more items you checked, the more you need my plan. So, let's get started before any more aging goes on!

Before you begin the actual diet I must first explain to you exactly what is happening to your body as you age and how that makes you fat. Then I'll set out a plan of action for you to allow you to reset your biological clock and start losing those excess pounds.

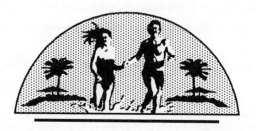

CHAPTER 2

Your Aging Metabolism

The first basic fact I want you to understand is that your age-related weight problem is not simply a matter of overeating. One thing that really galls me is the supercilious attitude of spouses, friends, and physicians who tell you, "The solution to your weight problem is simple. Just put down your fork and push yourself away from the table." This is simpleminded advice given by people who don't know what they are talking about.

These remarks are likely to make you feel guilty and blame your lack of willpower for your weight problem. Well, I can tell you that gaining weight as you grow older has nothing to do with willpower or lack of it. Neither is it caused by psychological problems. Depression, lack of self-esteem, anxiety, and feelings of inadequacy are the *results* of weight problems and not their cause.

The End of Your Guilt Trip

I'm going to put an end to your guilt trip right here and now. I never want you to feel guilty or self-conscious about your weight ever again. And don't listen to anyone who tells you that you should.

I'm not trying to provide you with excuses for your weight problem. I'm simply telling you that, as you get older, there are bodily factors at work that make it much more difficult for you to control your weight. Unless you understand what those factors are and how you can reverse their detrimental effects, you will remain overweight for the rest of your life. If you simply put the emphasis on "trying harder" to diet or removing the "psychological barriers" to weight loss, you will not only fail at permanently losing weight, you'll make yourself a nervous wreck in the process.

The main reason you have an age-related weight problem is because *your metabolism is getting old*. We must examine the reasons why it is aging and what we can do about it.

Metabolism and the 1949 Chevrolet

Let's first of all look at what is meant by the term *metabolism*. To understand this concept I want you to think of your body as an automobile and your metabolism as its engine.

Your metabolic engine works very hard. In fact, it never rests and is running 24 hours a day every day for your entire lifetime. When you are lying down or sleeping, your engine is idling. When you sit or stand, it's similar to pressing very lightly on your automobile's accelerator. When you walk around from one place to another you are pressing with more force. And there are times when you are jogging, cycling, or doing aerobic exercise that you are pressing your gas pedal all the way down to the floor.

The fuel or gasoline that your engine burns is analogous to the food that you eat. Gallons of gasoline can be compared to calories of food. In fact, a calorie is simply a unit measure of food energy.

Unlike your automobile engine, the more fuel your body's metabolic engine burns the better. You're not trying to conserve on caloric fuel, you're trying to burn up as much as possible, *especially when your engine is idling.*

Your engine burns calories in two ways. One is through *resting metabolism*, which refers to the amount of food energy your body uses just to keep your engine idling. In other words, this represents how many calories your body requires just to maintain life. The second is *movement metabolism*, which refers to how many calories your body uses through day-to-day activities and exercise.

It is important to realize that metabolism refers to a base rate of burning calories, as if your engine were idling all day long without your ever putting your foot down on the gas pedal. Think of this rate as the number of calories of food energy you would use up if you were lying down 24 hours a day without moving. In fact, it is this idling speed of your engine that we will be speeding up. As a result of the Hilton Head Over-35 Diet you will be burning more calories at rest, while you are lying down, sitting, and even while you are sleeping at night.

One other fact to consider is that if you were born in 1949, your body is like a 1949 Chevrolet. You were born as a 1949 Chevy and you will be driving that same car with that same engine for the rest of your life, perhaps until the year 2030 or later. As far as your body and its metabolism are concerned, you will never be able to trade it in for a new model.

You shouldn't be surprised that your metabolic engine

will require an occasional tune-up during your lifetime. In fact, unless periodic maintenance is performed, you might expect that your engine will become sluggish, erratic, and unreliable.

What Is Your Normal Idling Speed?

The speed of your resting metabolism is defined as *the number of calories your body burns at rest over a 24-hour period.* How your engine speed compares to someone else's is affected by a variety of factors such as heredity, body size, gender, past dieting history, and exercise level. The following chart indicates which of these factors helps and which hinders metabolic functioning.

Enhances Metabolism	Suppresses Metabolism
Slim parents	Fat parents
Tall, large frame	Short, small frame
Male	Female
Few diets in past	Many very low-cal or high-protein, low-carbohydrate diets in past
Regular exercise	Little exercise

As I discussed at length in my previous book, *The Hilton Head Metabolism Diet,* these factors along with others can combine to suppress your metabolism so it is burning at a much lower rate than it should be. By following my program, however, you can offset these factors and rev up your engine by 200, 300, or as many as 500 extra calories per day.

No matter what the rate of your metabolism based on

these individual factors, everybody's metabolism drops with age. To be more specific let's look at average metabolic rates and how they change with age. "Average" is difficult to define since so many factors influence a particular individual's metabolic rate. However, I have found that some women burn only 900 calories a day through metabolism while others burn as many as 1,500 calories a day. Men have a faster resting metabolism than women, ranging from 1,500 to 2,000 calories during each 24-hour period. Keep in mind that these are *resting* metabolic levels that do not include calories you would burn by exercising or by going through your day-to-day routine (especially if your responsibilities included a great deal of physical movement).

The Case of Ruth

Ruth is a 65-year-old widow from Florida who consulted me about her weight problem a year ago. She is a perky, outgoing person who loves to play bridge and enjoys traveling with her friends to exotic places around the world.

When my staff and I first evaluated her problem, Ruth weighed 172 pounds, much too much for a woman who was only 5-feet, 4-inches tall. At age 25 Ruth had weighed about 130 pounds and had maintained that weight through her late 30s. We calculated that during her younger years Ruth's body was burning approximately 1,450 calories a day through metabolism. Since she was a physically active person at that time (participating on a regular basis in swimming, walking, bicycling, and tennis) she was using up another 600 calories just by moving and exercising, allowing her to eat a total of 2,050 calories a day without gaining weight.

By age 65, the physiological effects of aging on her metabolism reduced her resting rate to 1,175 calories. Given her reduced level of physical activity with age, she now could eat only 1,350 *total* calories per day without running the risk of weight gain.

Since, on most days, she was eating slightly more than this amount, her body was storing those excess calories in the form of body fat. Since there are 3,500 calories in a pound of body fat, even eating 100 calories a day more than you are burning up will result in your gaining 12 extra pounds a year. Her older metabolism just could not keep up with the normal amount of food she was consuming.

Her doctor told her that she would have to reduce her food intake to 1,200 or 1,300 calories a day. Although Ruth tried this for a while, she found this restriction very difficult especially in view of all the traveling she did.

She read a magazine article about my work on metabolism and contacted me immediately. I am pleased to report that Ruth is back down to her 25-year-old weight of 130 pounds and after following the Hilton Head Over-35 Diet is now able to eat 1,800 calories a day without gaining an ounce. Needless to say she looks and feels like a new woman.

Can you imagine what age would do to your metabolic rate if, because of heredity or body size, you were on the low side of the metabolic range in your youth? By the time you are 50 you would have to follow a diet every day just to stay even with the few calories you are burning.

I definitely don't want you to do that. And, if you follow the Hilton Head Over-35 Diet, you won't have to. You'll be able to lead a normal life, eat a normal amount of food every day, and you will not have to be a slave to your aging metabolism.

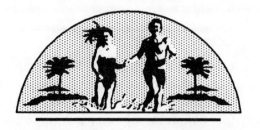

The Four Factors That Age Your Metabolism

Factor 1: Loss of Muscle Tissue

The prime culprit in metabolic sluggishness as you age is loss of muscle tissue. First of all, you should know that, while your body consists of many different kinds of tissue, from a metabolic standpoint we are most concerned with *fat* and *muscle* tissue. Fat or adipose tissue is relatively inert. That is, it just sits there in your body, not doing very much. At rest, it contributes very little to your overall resting metabolic rate. Muscle tissue, on the other hand, is physiologically active even at rest. It uses up many more calories of energy than does fat.

This is why, all other factors being equal, a muscular body burns more calories than a fat body. I'm not referring to how much you weigh but, rather, how much of that weight is muscle and how much is fat.

Lean body mass (a high proportion of muscle to fat) is

21

highly correlated with metabolic rate. If two people were identical in all respects, same body weight, same build, same sex, but one had more muscle tissue, that person would burn more calories each day, would be able to eat more without gaining weight, and would be able to lose weight faster on a diet.

Unfortunately, age takes its toll on lean body mass. As you reach your late 30s your muscle cells decrease in size and number. The physiology of your muscle changes so that the tissue eventually loses its capacity to regenerate new cells. However, with the Hilton Head Over-35 Diet you can slow down this process and stimulate the muscle fibers you have to their fullest.

Lost muscle tissue is often replaced by inert connective tissue or fat, both of which detract from your energy output. This loss of muscle tissue also contributes to a saggier, flabbier appearance. Simply put, your body starts to look older.

In addition to the aging process itself, your muscles can also atrophy and weaken through nonuse. If you become physically inactive with age your muscles simply won't develop as they once did.

Changes in your body composition with age actually begin at age 20. To give you a better idea of what I am talking about, here is what happens to your fat and muscle percentages as you get older:

Age	Muscle	Fat	Other
20	24%	15%	61%
40	20%	19%	61%
60	17%	23%	60%
70	13%	27%	60%

During the 50-year span between your 20th and your 70th birthdays, *you lose almost half of the muscle tissue in your body.* That's an astounding decline, especially since metabolic rate is so highly correlated with how much muscle you have. In fact, some experts believe that your lean body mass is the most important factor in determining the strength of your metabolism.

When evaluating this factor for clients at the Hilton Head Health Institute, we compute a ratio between fat weight and muscle or lean body mass. This ratio is expressed either as your *fat quotient* (percentage of body weight composed of fat) or your *lean body mass quotient* (percentage of weight composed of everything but fat).

Factor 2: Hormonal Changes: Your Aging Metabolism

Your metabolic rate is governed largely by your thyroid gland. The thyroid gland is located in the lower part of your neck and is shaped like a butterfly. It produces a hormone called thyroxine or T4. Thyroxine controls the rate at which chemical reactions occur in your body. If your thyroid does not produce enough thyroxine, your metabolism will be sluggish.

Your thyroid gland is controlled by the pituitary or "master" gland located at the base of your brain. It produces TSH or thyroid-stimulating hormone, which calls your thyroid gland into action. If your pituitary gland does not produce enough TSH, the result might also be a slower metabolism.

If your doctor suspected that your metabolism were sluggish due to a glandular abnormality, he or she would administer a blood test to check how much thyroxine is in your body. Your hormone level would be normal if the test showed that you had between 6 and 12 micrograms (a microgram is one-millionth of a gram) per 100 milliliters of blood. Before you go running to your doctor, let me remind you that 99 percent of overweight people have a normal amount of thyroxine in their bloodstream.

The important point to remember is that your metabolic rate can be sluggish without your having a medical problem with your glands. It could be that your thyroxine level is normal, but *low* normal. All this means is that your hormone output is lower than the average due to heredity, age, fad dieting, or several other factors.

Unfortunately, giving you thyroid tablets under these circumstances will not stimulate your thyroid to work harder. In fact, it is more likely that your thyroid gland will monitor this external source of T4 and produce *less* to compensate.

As you age, your glands simply aren't as efficient as they were in your youth. The chemical makeup of the cells in your body changes with age, resulting in less responsiveness to the hormones produced by your thyroid gland.

During periods of excitement, exertion, or stress, your adrenal glands (one located on top of each of your kidneys) secrete adrenaline or epinephrine, which increases your heart rate and metabolism for anywhere from one to three hours. Although this metabolic stimulation is relatively short-lived, you are still burning calories at a faster rate during these times. With age, the adrenal glands slow down, not responding as strongly or as quickly as they once did.

These age-related hormonal and cellular changes slow metabolic activity with each passing year.

Factor 3: Cellular Changes: Why Your Body Is Less Efficient in Transporting and Absorbing Nutrients

As you get older your body cannot transport or absorb the nutrients in the foods you eat as well as it once did. This is important from a weight-control standpoint because your metabolic engine functions best when it is fed a specific combination of nutrients.

Your metabolism is in high gear when you feed it a diet composed of 55–60 percent complex carbohydrates (fruits, vegetables, cereal, bread, potatoes, and pasta), 15–20 percent protein (milk, chicken, fish, legumes, nuts), and 25–30 percent fat (oil, salad dressing, butter). Eating these proportions of nutrients becomes even more crucial as you age, since the body cannot compensate for poor nutrition.

As you age there is a degeneration of the intestinal lining. As old cells in the intestinal wall wear out or die, your body lacks the capacity to regenerate new ones. Your cells are capable of dividing to form new cells only about 50 to 55 times during your lifetime. After that, many cells are unable to repair damage or replace themselves. Since nutrition is a crucial element in determining at what stage in your life your cells wear out, proper diet is extremely important in keeping you young.

In addition to the fact that your body does not absorb nutrients as well as it once did, transportation of nutrients through your bloodstream also becomes impaired. As you get older your blood vessels narrow, their walls thicken, and they become less elastic. The result is that fewer of the nutrients in the food you eat are distributed properly to the cells in your body.

This aging of your cells and blood vessels interferes with how many and what type of nutrients are available to feed your body. As a result your metabolic engine is shortchanged, not receiving the premium-quality fuel it requires for peak efficiency.

Research shows that in order to maintain a strong metabolism you must make certain that you eat an abundance (over half of your total calories) of complex carbohydrates. *It is especially critical for you to eat the right proportion of complex carbohydrates when you are over 35, since, because of the aging process, not all nutrients are transported or absorbed properly in your body.* You might have been able to get away with eating haphazardly when you were young, but not anymore. Now, unless you pay attention to fueling your metabolism correctly, you'll see the consequences next time you step on the scale.

Carbohydrates provide the long-term energy your body requires. When your body doesn't get enough carbohydrate from food, it is not able to produce enough glucose, a substance your cells need to function properly. When this happens, your body will convert the protein that you eat to carbohydrate in order to produce glucose. This is fine, up to a point. After a while, however, your body's protein needs increase since your protein is being converted to carbohydrate. This is the point at which your metabolism is really in danger, since your body goes right to the best source of protein you have—*muscle tissue*. That's right. Your body invades its own muscle and starts burning it up for energy. And you know what will happen next. Less muscle = a lower metabolism.

This is why it is so essential for you to follow the nutritional guidelines of the Hilton Head Over-35 Diet. It will provide you with the correct proportion of complex carbohydrates, protein, and fat that your over-35 body requires to compensate for the inefficiency of your aging cells.

Factor 4: Diminished Exercise Thermogenesis

If you are like most people over 35, you probably aren't as physically active as you once were. This may be due partly to a diminished inclination to exercise as you age and/or the fact that with your career, family, and social responsibilities, you simply can't find the time to exercise as regularly as you would like.

On the other hand, being less physically active than you once were can often be more directly related to aging itself.

With age, joints become less supple and, especially if you haven't been eating right, your stamina and endurance may be lacking. Many people come to the Institute with the complaint that back, knee, or joint problems that have worsened with age limit the intensity and amount of exercise they do.

Less physical activity causes muscle tissue gradually to atrophy. You actually lose muscle mass through disuse. And, since your muscle cells may have reached their 55-division lifetime maximum (even as early as middle age), you will have lost that muscle tissue forever. There goes your trim appearance and there goes your metabolism!

Regular physical activity also provides your resting metabolism with an extra boost through a process known as *exercise-induced thermogenesis*. Every time you take a walk or bike ride or swim a few laps your metabolic rate increases. In fact, once exercise charges up your engine, it stays charged up for hours after your exercise is over. This after-exercise boost is called thermogenesis.

I remember a client who, after going back home from the Institute, vowed to do to a one-hour brisk walk every morning. Five years later, this 46-year-old woman is still going strong, walking every morning at 7 A.M., rain or shine. We calculated that after each walk, her metabolism at rest ran a full 20 percent higher for the next three hours. This meant that even if she were sitting or lying down from 8 A.M. to 11 A.M., her metabolic engine was burning 20 percent more calories because of her walk earlier. Because of this thermogenic effect, she was burning an extra 12,000 calories a year *without moving*. That's 12,000 calories that you might *not* be burning by not exercising. Those 12,000 would be stored as fat somewhere on your body. *That's not even counting the calories saved or lost through the one-hour walk, just the thermogenic effect on resting metabolism after.*

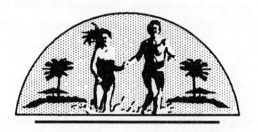

How Much Should You Weigh?

Before you begin the Hilton Head Over-35 Diet you must determine your current weight and then set a goal for your ideal weight. If you haven't already done so, weigh yourself on a reliable scale. If you have been overweight for a while you may have been avoiding the scale for fear of what it would tell you. One way of avoiding the fact that your weight is too high is to deny what is happening. Denial takes many forms—avoidance of the scale, not wanting to have your picture taken, refusing to discuss the issue with anyone. I can understand this defense mechanism, but the time for denial is over. This is the time to face your weight problem directly and overcome it.

Weigh yourself initially on whatever day you begin the Hilton Head Over-35 Diet. After that, follow my three rules of weighing:

RULE 1: Always weigh in the morning, as soon as you get out of bed.

RULE 2: Always weigh without clothes.

RULE 3: Only weigh *once a week on Friday morning.*

Rule 3 is especially important. At the beginning of a diet you will be tempted to weigh almost every day. You must resist this temptation. Focus your attention on following my diet and exercise plan and your weight will take care of itself. Because of changes in fat, muscle, and fluid in your body, once-a-week weighing gives you a much more accurate picture of your progress.

Weighing more than once a week is psychologically dangerous. If you haven't lost as much as you had expected (and expectations are almost always higher than what reality would dictate), you'll become upset and discouraged. Then you may either call it quits or change the diet in some way based on your superstitions of what might be keeping you from losing weight faster. For example, one woman told me that because her weight loss for the first week on my diet was "only" five pounds (which I consider very satisfactory), she decided to eat only half of the food that I prescribe. She was flabbergasted when, over the next few days, she didn't lose any weight at all. I explained to her that by eating less than the diet requires she was actually slowing down her metabolism and burning fewer calories. In addition, she had changed the nutritional balance of the diet so that her body was probably starting to burn muscle tissue as well as fat.

You must not change any element of my system because of an emotional response to the scale. You must not allow your scale to have that much influence over you.

Since you will be weighing yourself only once a week, I suggest you put your scale in a closet or in a cabinet until you are ready to weigh yourself. If it is sitting out in your bathroom, you will surely be tempted to weigh.

I remember a woman at the Institute who, after her first

weigh-in, asked us not to tell her how much weight she had lost each week. She knew she had a tendency to overreact in a negative way to her weight losses (even if they were good) and she was determined not to let this reaction influence her motivation. Since she had to lose 75 pounds, she continued losing weight at home after spending four weeks at the Institute. She successfully lost all of her weight even though *she did not weigh herself on a scale one time during the five months that it took her to lose her weight.* Now, that's willpower! She knew she had finally reached her goal by her clothing size and body measurements.

Enough said about weighing.

Let's set a goal weight for you by finding out how much you should weigh. When I say *should* weigh I am referring to a *healthy*, trim weight. The following charts (developed in 1983 by the Metropolitan Life Insurance Company) will help you determine an ideal weight based on your height and body frame.

To determine whether you have a small, medium, or large frame, measure the *size of your elbow*, using the following procedure:

1. Extend your right arm straight out in front of your body. Hold your hand open with your palm facing upward.
2. Bend your forearm upward at a 90-degree angle.
3. Place the thumb and index finger of your other hand on either side of your bent elbow. Make sure your thumb and finger are resting on the two prominent bones in your elbow.
4. Pull your thumb and finger away slightly, just barely maintaining contact with your elbow. Make certain you keep the same spacing between your fingers.
5. Have someone measure the space between your thumb and finger.

IDEAL BODY WEIGHTS FOR WOMEN

Height	Small Frame	Medium Frame	Large Frame
4'10"	102–111	109–121	118–131
4'11"	103–113	111–123	120–134
5' 0"	104–115	113–126	122–137
5' 1"	106–118	115–129	125–140
5' 2"	108–121	118–132	128–143
5' 3"	111–124	121–135	131–147
— 5' 4"—	114–127	—124–138—	134–151
5' 5"	117–130	127–141	137–155
5' 6"	120–133	130–144	140–159
5' 7"	123–136	133–147	143–163
5' 8"	126–139	136–150	147–167
5' 9"	129–142	139–153	149–170
5'10"	132–145	142–156	152–173
5'11"	135–148	145–159	155–176
6' 0"	138–151	148–162	158–179

6. Use the charts on pages 33 and 34 and compare your elbow measurement with those listed for the small, medium, and large categories.

Now that you know your frame size, find the appropriate ideal weight range for your height. Since these are fairly wide ranges, your exact ideal weight will depend on two factors:

1. The weight at which you feel physically and psychologically the best
2. The weight within that range that is easiest for you to maintain

First of all, you must be satisfied with how you look and feel at a particular weight. If I told you that you would be

IDEAL BODY WEIGHTS FOR MEN

Height	Small Frame	Medium Frame	Large Frame
5' 2"	128–134	131–141	138–150
5' 3"	130–136	133–143	140–153
5' 4"	132–138	135–145	142–156
5' 5"	134–140	137–148	144–160
5' 6"	136–142	139–151	146–164
5' 7"	138–145	142–154	149–168
5' 8"	140–148	145–157	152–172
5' 9"	142–151	148–160	155–176
5'10"	144–154	151–163	158–180
5'11"	146–157	154–166	161–184
6' 0"	149–160	157–170	164–188
6' 1"	152–164	160–174	168–192
6' 2"	155–168	164–178	172–197
6' 3"	158–172	167–182	176–202
6' 4"	162–176	171–187	181–207

BODY FRAME SIZES FOR WOMEN
BASED ON ELBOW MEASUREMENT

Height	Small Frame	Medium Frame	Large Frame
4'10"—5' 3"	Less than 2¼"	2¼"—2½"	More than 2½"
5' 4"—5'11"	Less than 2⅜"	2⅜"—2⅝"	More than 2⅝"
6' 0"—up	Less than 2½"	2½"—2¾"	More than 2¾"

BODY FRAME SIZES FOR MEN
BASED ON ELBOW MEASUREMENT

Height	Small Frame	Medium Frame	Large Frame
5'2"—5'3"	Less than 2½"	2½"—2⅞"	More than 2⅞"
5'4"—5'7"	Less than 2⅝"	2⅝"—2⅞"	More than 2⅞"
5'8"—5'11"	Less than 2¾"	2¾"—3"	More than 3"
6'0"—6'3"	Less than 2¾"	2¾"—3⅛"	More than 3⅛"
6'4"—up	Less than 2⅞"	2⅞"—3¼"	More than 3¼"

healthy and trim weighing 135 pounds but you like your appearance better at 130 pounds, so be it. You may even find that five pounds one way or the other is significant in terms of clothing sizes. A particular woman might fit more easily into a size 8 dress at 130 pounds and find that she is between sizes at 135 pounds. You may also find that the overall feel of your body is more acceptable to you at one weight as opposed to another.

A second consideration is that you may find that some body weights are easier to maintain than others. Sometimes only five or six pounds can make the world of difference between a struggle over calories and a more relaxed approach to maintenance. This is due to the fact that your body has a *set point*, a weight at which it is most biologically comfortable. If that set point is close to your charted ideal weight range you can simply choose one weight over another to make things easy on yourself. However, if your set point is much higher than your ideal range, you are going to have to fight your biological setting and keep your weight within the healthier range. Keep in mind that the Hilton Head Over-35 Diet is designed to lower the setting on your biological weight-thermostat to bring it in line with your healthy, ideal weight.

In any event I would suggest you choose an ideal range of five pounds instead of one particular number. That is, a man who is 5 feet, 10 inches tall with a medium frame might choose to maintain an ideal weight between 158 and 163 pounds as opposed to saying he will weigh exactly 160 pounds for the rest of his life.

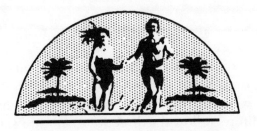

How Fast
Is Your Metabolic
Engine?

Most people have no idea how many calories their metabolic engines burn each day. I'm going to show you how to figure out the strength of your individual metabolism. Although these tests involve a series of mathematical calculations, please bear with me. I will take you through the process one step at a time and make it easy for you. The knowledge you gain from these tests will be worthwhile, especially later in the book, when I discuss how to maintain your weight loss.

We will be determining both your *resting metabolic rate* and your *total calorie expenditure* per day. Resting rate refers to the number of calories your body burns *at rest* (with no body movement at all) just to maintain life. Total expenditure equals the number of calories you burn through metabolism *and* movement and exercise. This is the most important factor since it will indicate the number of calories you can eat without putting on weight.

Before we find your resting metabolic rate and total calorie expenditure, follow the directions below to calculate your Weight Factor, Height Factor, and Age Factor. These factors are required for the metabolic formula that will tell us what we want to know.

Please note there are different procedures for men and women.

Weight, Height, and Age Factors for Women

To Find Your Weight Factor:

- Multiply your ideal weight in pounds by .45. *Make certain this is a weight in your ideal range and not your current weight.*
- Multiply the resulting number by 9.56.
- The number is your Weight Factor. 636.70

EXAMPLE **Betty's ideal weight is 124 pounds. We multiply it by .45 and obtain 55.80. We then multiply this number by 9.56 to find Betty's Weight Factor of 533.45.**

To Find Your Height Factor:

- Multiply your height in inches by 2.5.
- Multiply the resulting number by 1.85.
- This number is your Height Factor.

EXAMPLE **Betty is 5 feet, 4 inches tall, which converts to 64 inches. We multiply 64 by 2.5 and get 160. We then multiply 160 by 1.85 to find her Height Factor of 296.**

To Find Your Age Factor:

- Multiply your age by 4.68.
- This number is your Age Factor.

EXAMPLE **Betty is 45 years of age. When we multiply 45 by 4.68 we find that Betty's Age Factor is 210.60.**

Weight, Height, and Age Factors for Men

To Find Your Weight Factor:

- Multiply your ideal weight in pounds by .45. *Make certain this is a weight in your ideal range and not your current weight.*
- Multiply the resulting number by 13.5.
- This number is your Weight Factor.

EXAMPLE **Joe's ideal weight is 160 pounds. When we multiply 160 by .45 we obtain 72. We then multiply 72 by 13.5 to find Joe's Weight Factor of 972.**

To Find Your Height Factor:

- Multiply your height in inches by 2.5.
- Multiply the resulting number by 5.
- This number is your Height Factor.

EXAMPLE **Joe is 5 feet, 9 inches tall, which converts into 69 inches. When we multiply 69 by 2.5 we get 172.50. By multiplying 172.50 by 5 we obtain a Height Factor for Joe of 862.50.**

To Find Your Age Factor:

- Multiply your age by 6.75.
- This number is your Age Factor. *50625*

EXAMPLE **Joe is 40 years of age. When we multiply 40
by 6.75 we find Joe's Age Factor to be 270.**

Now you are ready to do a little addition and subtraction
to find your *Resting Metabolic Rate*. Once again, notice there
are different formulas for men and women.

Resting Metabolic Rate for Women

- Add your Weight Factor to 655.1.
- Add your Height Factor to the answer.
- Subtract your Age Factor from the answer.
- The resulting number is your Resting Metabolic Rate per
  day.

EXAMPLE **Betty's Weight Factor is 533.45. We add this
number to 655.1 to obtain 1,188.55. We then
add 1,188.55 to Betty's Height Factor of 296.
This gives us 1,484.55. We then subtract Betty's
Age Factor of 210.60 from 1,484.55 which
gives us 1,273.95. To simplify matters we'll
round this number off to 1,274. This is Betty's
Resting Metabolic Rate.**

Resting Metabolic Rate for Men

- Add your Weight Factor to 66.5.
- Add your Height Factor to the answer.
- Subtract your Age Factor from the answer.

• The resulting number is your Resting Metabolic Rate per day.

EXAMPLE   Joe's Weight Factor is 972. We add this number to 66.5 to obtain 1,038.50. We then add Joe's Height Factor of 862.50 to 1,038.50 to get 1901. Next, we subtract Joe's Age Factor of 270 from 1,901 which gives us 1,631. This means that Joe's Resting Metabolic Rate is 1,631 calories per day.

Because there are individual differences in metabolic rate based on heredity, your metabolism may actually be 15 percent lower than this figure. Because of this fact, it is better to establish a range for your metabolism, indicating the minimum number of calories you might burn as well as the maximum number.

To find your minimum metabolic level, multiply your Resting Metabolic Rate by .85. For example, if we multiply Betty's rate of 1,274 by .85 we would find that her minimum resting metabolic rate would be 1,083 calories a day. This indicates that her probable resting metabolic range would be from 1,083 to 1,274 calories a day.

This Resting Metabolic Rate is the number of calories your body burns at rest during each 24-hour time period. For women, this number ranges between 900 and 1,600 calories per day. Men have metabolic rates ranging from 1,200 to 1,900 calories a day. Where your metabolism falls along this range is, to a large extent, a function of your age and how much muscle you have lost through the aging process.

Because you are moving about during the day, the total calories your body burns in a 24-hour period is higher than your metabolic rate. Obviously, the more you move around and the more you exercise, the more total calories you will burn. If you were bedridden for a few days because of an illness or hospitalization, you would not be burning many more calories than your metabolic rate. Therefore, you would not be able to eat very much without gaining weight. If more calories are being consumed than are being burned, your body stores those extra calories as fat. Every time these excess calories add up to 3,500, you have gained a pound.

To determine total caloric expenditure, multiply your minimum and maximum metabolic rate by one of the following numbers, depending on your level of physical activity:

Multiply by:	If your activity is:
1.3	Very Light
1.5	Light
1.6	Moderate
1.9	Heavy

If you do not engage in regularly scheduled exercise such as walking, aerobic dance, jogging, or bicycling several times a week, consider yourself to be in the Very Light to Light categories. The difference between these categories is related to the amount of moving around you do during the day. If you are sitting or lying down most of the time, even if you are busy, you would be in the Very Light activity category.

Betty's resting metabolic range fell between 1,083 and 1,274 calories and she is in the Light Activity category. When we multiply her minimum and maximum metabolic rates by 1.5, we obtain the following answer:

Total Caloric Expenditure Range = 1,625–1,911

This means that, once Betty loses her weight, she will be able to maintain her ideal weight by eating between 1,625 and 1,911 calories each day. Of course, the moderate exercise program I will prescribe will put both you and Betty in the Heavy-Moderate activity category, which will give you even more calories to eat.

Let's Get Started

Now that you have a good indication of your weight goal and metabolic rate, it's time to get started with the Hilton Head Over-35 Diet. As you continue with the program you should weigh yourself every Friday to keep up with your progress.

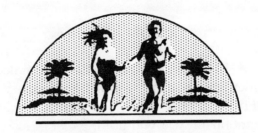

Getting Started: The Five Essential Rules of the Hilton Head Over-35 Diet

Medical Advice

When beginning this or any other diet or exercise program, it is advisable to consult your personal physician. He or she may wish to give you a medical evaluation or to advise you in specific ways. This is particularly true if you are over 45 years of age or if you have any one of the following characteristics:

- High blood pressure
- Elevated cholesterol
- Cigarette smoker
- Diabetes
- Family history of heart disease
- Orthopedic problems.

Since the Hilton Head Over-35 Diet is designed especially for your older metabolism, it will be necessary for you to follow my Five Essential Rules. Remember, because of your sluggish metabolism, you will not be able to lose weight *and* rejuvenate your metabolic rate simply by reducing your calories. Just any diet will not work for you.

You must realize that being overweight is merely a symptom of your more basic metabolic problem. You require a special program designed just for you.

Think of my Five Essential Rules as a prescription given to you by your doctor. If your doctor tells you that, to cure your disease, you must take five pills a day, do you only take two or three? Of course not. My rules, just like medicine, contain the essential ingredients to rid you of your weight problem.

ESSENTIAL RULE 1: You Must Eat Four to Five Times a Day

This rule may seem a little odd at first. Imagine me telling you that the way to lose weight is to eat more often instead of less. But that's exactly what your metabolism needs. Unfortunately, in the past, you may have been skipping meals to lose weight. Without realizing it you were actually suppressing your metabolism by doing this.

You should eat more times each day because of a metabolic process known as *dietary thermogenesis* or, more simply, the *thermic effect*. Thermogenesis literally refers to an increase in the body's heat production, essentially, an increase in metabolic rate. The thermic effect occurs every time you eat a meal and it results in your burning more calories for two to three hours after you have eaten. At its peak, thermogenesis boosts your metabolism as much as 40 percent above its normal level.

In real terms, this means that your resting metabolic rate

is increased by about 10–15 percent for two to three hours after every meal. Even if you were sitting or lying down during that time your body would still be burning 10–15 percent more calories than it would have if you hadn't eaten.

Let's suppose that two women, Jill and Barbara, each went on a diet. Both women have a metabolic rate of 1,900 calories per day. Jill never eats breakfast, skips lunch to try to save calories, and eats dinner at 6:30 P.M. Her total extra burn-off from her one thermic effect during the day is only 36 calories. Barbara, on the other hand, divides her calories into five meals a day, two mini-meals in addition to breakfast, lunch, and dinner. Just by eating more often Barbara burns an extra 178 calories a day above and beyond her resting metabolic level. This may not seem like a lot but, believe me, it adds up fast. In Barbara's case, thermogenesis would help burn more than 65,000 extra calories a year!

Not only will the thermic effect help you lose more weight while on the Hilton Head Over-35 Diet but it will help you keep that weight off for the rest of your life. By eating five times a day at maintenance, you would avoid gaining 18 pounds a year. It's quite amazing how easy it is to burn calories once you understand some of the basic mechanisms governing your metabolism.

The strength of the dietary-thermogenesis reaction is related to fat-versus-lean body-mass ratio. The more muscle and the less fat you have, the more thermogenesis you experience after meals. Unfortunately, what this means is that those who need to burn the extra calories the most, experience the thermal effect the least. It also means that, as you lose muscle tissue through aging and inactivity, thermogenesis is of less and less benefit to your metabolism.

The good news for you is that as you lose fat and increase your lean body mass through the Hilton Head Over-35 Diet, you will benefit even more from thermogenesis. That will help you keep your weight off once you've lost your excess pounds.

The Metabo-Meal

To take advantage of this bodily reaction to food, the Hilton Head Over-35 Diet provides you with three main meals each day plus one mini-meal on weekdays and two mini-meals on weekends. These mini-meals are called *Metabo-Meals* (pronounce with an emphasis on "tab").
Your meals will be divided as follows:

Weekdays	Weekends
Breakfast	Breakfast
Lunch	Lunch
Metabo-Meal	Metabo-Meal
Dinner	Dinner
	Metabo-Meal

People who eat dinner early (between 5 P.M. and 6 P.M.) during the week have the option of eating their Metabo-Meal in the evening, between 8:30 P.M. and 9:30 P.M.
As you will see in a later chapter, the Metabo-Meals consist of a relatively small amount of food such as a bowl of cereal or a piece of fruit. While you might consider these to be snacks I would prefer that you think of them as meals. The word *snack* has a negative connotation. Meals, on the other hand, even mini-meals, are essential nutrition for your body.

ESSENTIAL RULE 2: You Must Exercise After Meals

With this rule I am again challenging a long-standing taboo. You may have heard at some time in your life that strenuous exercise after a large meal is not good for you, that it puts too much stress on the body. It is true, in fact, that after eating a meal, more blood and oxygen are sent to your stomach and intestines so your body can begin to digest the food. Because of this, if you do very strenuous exercise after a large meal, you may experience muscle cramping in your legs or arms since the oxygen your muscles need for this activity is being diverted elsewhere.

The key phrases to remember here are *large meal* and *strenuous exercise*. Certainly you should not go out and run five miles at top speed after you have just eaten a 1,000-calorie meal. On the other hand, moderate exercise such as walking after a small to moderate-sized meal is not at all harmful, and, in fact, is actually beneficial for your metabolism.

Researchers have found that a relationship exists between dietary thermogenesis and exercise. Moderately paced exercise after a meal will *double* the number of extra calories by which the thermic effect increases your metabolism. This means that exercise after a meal is worth more calories than it is at any other time during the day. For example, you are practically supercharging your metabolism by taking a walk *after* breakfast instead of walking before you eat in the morning.

Exercise after meals not only increases the strength of the thermic effect but also makes it last longer. By eating a meal and exercising afterward your resting metabolic rate is boosted by 20–25 percent for the next three to four hours. Just think of all those pounds melting away!

The Thermal Walk

In order to use these research results to stimulate your metabolism, the diet includes two *thermal walks* a day. A thermal walk is simply an after-meal walk that is moderately paced. I'll give you more details on speed and distance later. For now, just get ready for a 40-minute morning thermal walk after breakfast and a shorter 20-minute thermal walk after any other meal (including your Metabo-Meals) during the day. I realize that I'm asking for a total of an hour out of your busy schedule, but walking is a must if you are to successfully rejuvenate your metabolism.

These thermal walks will stimulate metabolic activity and burn more calories than any equivalent exercise you've ever done before. However, if you are very overweight, have to lose over fifty pounds, or have an orthopedic or cardiac problem, you should consult your physician before beginning this thermal walk program.

ESSENTIAL RULE 3: **You Must Eat More Calories on Weekends Than You Do During the Week**

One of the facts we have learned about metabolism over the years is that when you lower your caloric intake in order to lose weight, your metabolism has a tendency to slow down. Just when you are trying to burn more calories your body wants to burn fewer. This is certainly a dilemma that we must counteract.

This paradox is explained by the fact that your body is built for survival, not dieting. When you drastically reduce the number of calories you eat, an alarm system goes off in your body. This is your survival alarm. Your body is now on guard for the potential of starvation. Of course, you are not starving, you are dieting. But your body has no way of telling the difference.

Because of this, your body tries to "save your life" by conserving energy, by slowing down all metabolic processes, and so your metabolism is put in slow motion. If you were really starving, this reaction might save you from starving to death or at least postpone the inevitable.

This lowering of your metabolic rate continues as long as you stay on your diet. This is why you may have found that on past diets you lose more weight in the first two weeks than you do later in the diet. As long as you are dieting (whether you are eating 800 calories or 1,200 calories), your metabolism continues on its downward course. Unless something is done, you could end up burning 25 percent fewer calories a day. This, however, is the last thing we want to happen.

Unless we counteract this metabolic decline, it can also cause problems after you lose your weight. When you start eating normally again, you will have a tendency to put weight back on since your metabolism is not burning many calories. Although with normal eating your metabolism will eventually revive itself, you can't afford to wait for this readjustment to occur naturally. You must take steps right from the beginning of the diet to keep your metabolism strong now—and to sustain its high level after you lose your weight.

Another interesting fact about metabolism provides us with an answer to this problem: Just as your metabolic rate is suppressed in response to fewer calories, it is also stimulated when calories are increased. But you obviously can't simply eat a lot more calories and expect to lose weight. So I have devised a system by which we can periodically stimulate your metabolism with more calories but maintain your rate of weight loss at the same time.

The Booster Weekend

The optimum solution lies in varying your calories so that you eat a low number of calories during the week and more calories each weekend. You continue to alternate between the Low-Cal Weekdays and the Booster Weekend. The Booster Weekend provides 300 more calories and one extra meal. As you will see later, these calories are spread out throughout the day so you eat slightly more food at every meal. These extra calories boost your metabolic rate without causing your weight loss to slow down.

If you are familiar with my previous book, *The Hilton Head Metabolism Diet,* you will remember that I advocated a two-week Low Cal/one-week Booster alternation. The Booster

Weekend strategy is more effective, particularly for those over 35 years of age.

A side benefit to the Booster Weekend is that it provides more flexibility to your diet on the weekends. The extra calories allow you to entertain or eat out on Saturday and Sunday with more ease.

ESSENTIAL RULE 4: You Must Eat Mostly Grain-Based Foods, Starches, Vegetables, and Fruit

As I mentioned earlier, your metabolism functions best when it is fed an abundance of *complex carbohydrates*. These nutrients include grain-based foods (cereal and bread), starches (potatoes, pasta), vegetables, and fruit. These foods not only stimulate your metabolism but they also provide energy.

Complex carbohydrates constitute the best fuel for your metabolism for two reasons. First, they reduce the tendency of your body to lower your metabolic rate when you decrease food intake. This automatic conservation of calories in response to dieting is much less pronounced on a regimen of complex carbohydrates. These foods keep your metabolism strong and, along with my exercise program, will offset your body's "starvation" response. Diets high in protein or very low in daily calories (from 400 to 600) have the opposite effect; they push your metabolism to an abnormally low level.

The second reason complex carbohydrates help strengthen your metabolism is that they preserve muscle tissue. When you go on low-complex-carbohydrate diets your body loses muscle as well as fat as part of your total weight loss. To keep your metabolism energized we must prevent this at all costs. You are losing enough muscle tissue through the aging process. You certainly don't want to accelerate this loss by eating the wrong foods.

Of course your metabolism also requires protein and fat as part of its overall fuel. The Hilton Head Over-35 Diet provides you with the exact combination of nutrients that your metabolism needs. Your optimum metabolic fuel consists of:

60 percent Complex Carbohydrates
15 percent Protein
25 percent Fat

You won't have to bother yourself with calculating how many calories of carbohydrates, protein, and fat you are eating because I have figured this out for you in advance. All you have to do is follow the menu plans and you will be eating the correct food for your metabolism. I don't even want you to have to count calories, so that's all been arranged also. You have more important things to do, so I have made the diet as easy as possible for you to follow without disrupting your life.

Because the diet is designed to keep you healthy as well as slim, you will be asked to reduce your intake of sugar, salt, and fat. Your over-35 body has increasing difficulty in processing blood sugar. Such glucose intolerance can lead to diabetes and even an increased level of fats in your blood that could contribute to atherosclerosis (a narrowing of the arteries caused by a build-up of plaque) and heart disease. While the diet will temporarily eliminate sweets, once you lose your weight, you will be able to eat them in moderation. In fact, physiological improvements resulting from this diet will actually help your body metabolize sugar more effectively.

As you probably know, excessive salt intake is associated with high blood pressure and fluid retention. The Hilton Head Over-35 Diet is a low-sodium diet that gives you no more than 1,500 to 2,000 milligrams of sodium per day. To keep your sodium level under control you will be asked not to add salt to your food during cooking or at the table. Even if you don't add any, you will be getting more than enough sodium for your body simply through the foods you will be eating.

You will also be asked to take a vitamin/mineral supplement while on the diet to provide your body with everything it needs to fight the aging process. Women will be instructed to take a calcium supplement to help prevent osteoporosis (a thinning of the bones that occurs with age).

Specific guidelines will be provided with the daily meal plans.

ESSENTIAL RULE 5: **You Must Strengthen Your Muscle Tissue Three Times a Week**

In order to stimulate and rejuvenate your metabolism you must not only lose fat but, even more important, you must gain muscle tissue. As you know by now, the more muscle you have, the stronger is your metabolic rate.

Thermal walks burn calories and strengthen leg and buttocks muscles. However, thermal walks must be supplemented with exercises that strengthen the muscles in the upper portion of your body. These *muscle reconditioners* will not only stimulate your metabolism but also contour your body to give it a firm, youthful look. After just a few weeks of reconditioning your muscles you'll be amazed at how much younger you look and feel.

These muscle reconditioners require only 20 minutes, three times a week. They don't even add to your overall physical activity time since you will be doing them after a meal, in place of your 20-minute thermal walk, three days a week.

Let's Get More Specific

Now that you understand my Five Essential Rules, let's review them:

ESSENTIAL RULE 1: **You Must Eat Four to Five Times a Day**

ESSENTIAL RULE 2: **You Must Exercise After Meals**

ESSENTIAL RULE 3: **You Must Eat More Calories on Weekends Than You Do During the Week**

ESSENTIAL RULE 4: **You Must Eat Mostly Grain-Based Foods, Starches, Vegetables, and Fruit**

ESSENTIAL RULE 5: **You Must Strengthen Your Muscle Tissue Three Times a Week**

Now it's time for my step-by-step plan of action to enable you to implement these rules. The first phase of the Hilton Head Over-35 Diet will be the Low-Cal Weekday Menu Plan.

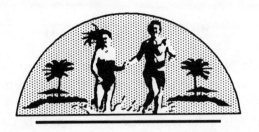

CHAPTER 7

Low-Cal Weekday Menu Plan

You should follow this plan from Monday through Friday. The foods are simple and easy to prepare. Although the meals are designed to keep preparation time to a minimum, I have included recipes of special dishes we serve at the Hilton Head Health Institute for you to try when you have the time or inclination.

Vitamin/Mineral Supplement

Before starting the Hilton Head Over-35 Diet you must first purchase a good multivitamin/mineral supplement. Based on your needs as an over-35 individual I have found that commercial vitamins that give you close to 100 percent of the recommended daily allowances for vitamins are the best. Your pharmacist will be able to provide choices for you.

Take one of these a day until you lose your weight. After that, if you are eating according to the maintenance guidelines, you will not require any extra vitamins or minerals.

I might also note that most of the cereals I recommend are fortified with vitamins and minerals and many provide a good percentage of your requirements for the day.

Calcium Supplement for Women

In addition to the vitamin/mineral supplement, women require an extra dose of calcium. Actually, this is not only required while dieting but for the rest of your life to help slow down the aging of your bones. Most experts agree that the time to start calcium supplements is when you are 35 years of age.

Prior to menopause, women need up to 1,000–1,200 milligrams of calcium per day. Postmenopausal women need up to 1,500 milligrams a day unless they are undergoing estrogen therapy to slow bone loss, in which case they may need only 1,000 milligrams.

Since the Hilton Head Over-35 Diet will be providing natural sources of calcium (primarily from milk, cheese, and leafy green vegetables), you will need to supplement your calcium intake by only 500 milligrams per day. Premenopausal women should take two 250-milligram tablets of calcium a day. If you are past menopause you will require two 500-milligram tablets per day. Your body uses calcium more efficiently if you spread out the dose, taking one tablet in the morning and one in the evening.

There are many over-the-counter calcium supplements on the market containing various forms of calcium. Probably the best supplement is in the form of calcium carbonate because it contains the highest concentration of calcium and is relatively inexpensive.

In any event, *you should consult your physician before taking any calcium supplements.* A small minority of people (for example, those with a history of kidney stones) must be careful about excess calcium.

Basic Guidelines for the Hilton Head Over-35 Diet

- Drink plenty of fluid (at least four eight-ounce glasses of liquid a day). Make sure that all of the liquids you drink are noncaloric and that most are decaffeinated. Caffeine in coffee, tea, and soft drinks is a diuretic, robbing your body of the fluid it needs. Your body will be losing fluid on the diet and you must replace it to help you metabolize, transport, and absorb nutrients properly.
- Avoid alcoholic beverages. They contain "empty" calories and you will not lose weight as fast if you drink them. You can drink again in moderation after you lose your weight.
- Do not add salt to your food during cooking or at the table. Salt substitutes are unnecessary and might aggravate your salt cravings.
- You may add herbs and spices to any food. Just make certain that any commercial herb/spice mixes you use do not contain sodium.
- Remove all visible fat from meats and remove the skin from chicken before eating it.
- Buy only fresh or frozen vegetables and fruits. *Never* buy canned.
- Never add sauces, butter, etc., to main course or vegetable dishes unless specified.
- Buy one to two ounces more of the fish, chicken, and

beef portions indicated in the menu plan. The reason for this is that the portions listed refer to *cooked* ounces and you must allow for shrinkage during cooking.
- Eat only what the menu plan instructs. Substitutions should occur only occasionally.

When You Should Eat Your Meals

As you know, you will be eating four times a day—breakfast, lunch, dinner, and Metabo-Meal. Feel free to fit these meals into your normal schedule during the day. However, try to allow at least three hours between any two meals. If you eat dinner later than 6:30 P.M. it is permissible to eat your Metabo-Meal in the mid to late afternoon. The most important thing for you to keep in mind is that *you must eat all of the meals and all of the food prescribed.* If you modify the diet your metabolism will not be receiving the proper fuel to keep it strong and you will not experience the desired results.

How These Menus Differ from the Hilton Head Metabolism Diet

If you are familiar with my previous book, *The Hilton Head Metabolism Diet*, you will notice three major differences in this new menu plan. First, the Over-35 Diet has a different nutritional balance than the Metabolism Diet, featuring more complex-carbohydrate foods for metabolic stimulation. Second, the Over-35 Diet offers a greater range of food choices and more varied recipes. Third, calories in the Over-35 Diet are distributed among the meals differently, so that more food is eaten earlier in the day. All of these changes are the result of research at the Hilton Head Health Institute and are designed to further increase metabolic rate.

Low-Cal Menus

Below are Low-Cal Menus for three weeks. If your weight requires you to stay on the diet for a longer period of time, simply repeat this three-week cycle (using the recipes in Appendix A for variety) until you reach your ideal weight. Remember, you should eat Low-Cal Menus from Monday through Friday. Booster Weekend Menus for Saturday and Sunday are described in the next chapter.

W E E K 1

Breakfast Every Weekday:

Cereal (¾ cup)—choice of Special K, Raisin Bran, Just Right, Product 19, Nutri-Grain, ProGrain, corn flakes, shredded wheat, oatmeal (cooked)
Milk (½ cup)—low-fat (2 percent) or skim only
Fruit (½ piece)—choice of orange, banana, grapefruit, peach, pear, apple (or ¼ medium cantaloupe or ⅛ medium honeydew)
Coffee or tea—sugar substitute and/or dash of low-fat or skim milk may be added, if desired

M O N D A Y

Breakfast:

Low-cal breakfast as prescribed

Lunch:

Turkey Sandwich:
  Turkey (1 ounce slice)
  Low-cal mayonnaise (1 teaspoon)

Tomato (2 slices)
Lettuce (1 medium leaf)
Low-calorie wheat bread (2 slices)
Fruit/Yogurt Mix (mix ¼ cup strawberries with 2 ounces plain, low-fat yogurt)

Dinner:

Baked fish (5 ounces cooked with 1 tablespoon lemon juice/1 teaspoon diet margarine combination)
Roasted Chips (½ potato)—see recipe in Appendix A
Green beans (½ cup)

Metabo-Meal:

Seedless grapes (½ cup)

T U E S D A Y

Breakfast:

Low-cal breakfast as prescribed

Lunch:

Primavera Salad 1½ cups (Pasta/vegetable combination)—see recipe in Appendix A

Dinner:

Pork Tenderloin (3 ounces)
Carrots (½ cup, diced)
New potatoes (3 medium-size)

Metabo-Meal:

Cereal (¾ cup Special K, Corn Flakes, or Product 19)
Milk (½ cup skim or 2 percent low-fat)

W E D N E S D A Y

Breakfast:

Low-cal breakfast as prescribed

Lunch:

Pita Sandwich:
Pita bread (1)
Tuna salad (1 ounce)—see recipe in Appendix A
Tomato (½ cup chopped)
Onion (1 tablespoon, chopped)
Lettuce (¾ cup lettuce, chopped)

195

Dinner:

Choice of Jamaican Chicken, Mexican Chicken, or Chicken Cacciatore (1 breast)—see recipes in Appendix A
Rice (¼ cup)
Broccoli (½ cup)

180

Metabo-Meal

Apple (1 medium to large)

T H U R S D A Y

Breakfast:

Low-cal breakfast as prescribed

Lunch:

Spinach and Mushroom Omelet—see recipe in Appendix A
Low-cal whole-wheat bread (1 slice)
Dessert:
Cantaloupe (¼)

Dinner:

Lasagna—see recipe in Appendix A
Garden salad (small tossed salad with lettuce, tomato, radishes, and 1 tablespoon low-cal dressing)

Metabo-Meal:

Popcorn (4 cups of air-popped; no butter or salt)

F R I D A Y

Breakfast:

Low-cal breakfast as prescribed

Lunch:

Large tossed salad:
    Lettuce (2 cups of iceberg, Bibb, or romaine)
    Tomato (1, sliced or diced)
    Onion rings (3)

Green pepper rings (2)
Low-cal salad dressing (2 tablespoons)
Dessert:
Pear (1, cut in wedges)

Dinner:

Boiled shrimp (5 ounces)
Cocktail sauce (2 tablespoons of commercial sauce)
Corn on the cob (1 medium ear with 2 teaspoons diet
  margarine)
Hawaiian Cole Slaw (¾ cup)—see recipe in Appendix A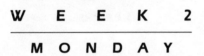

Metabo-Meal

Cereal (¾ cup of any of the prescribed breakfast cereals)
Milk (½ cup skim or 2 percent low-fat)

S A T U R D A Y   A N D   S U N D A Y

• *Refer to the next chapter for booster weekend menu plans.*

W E E K   2

M O N D A Y

Breakfast:

Low-cal breakfast as prescribed

Lunch:

Spinach Salad:
  Fresh spinach (2 cups)
  Mushrooms (½ cup)

Onion rings (5)
Hard-boiled egg (1, sliced)
Tomato (1 medium, sliced or diced)
Low-cal salad dressing (2 tablespoons)
Melba toast (2)

Dinner:

Rock Cornish hen (1 whole, 16-ounce size; yields 5 ounces
    cooked meat)
Curried Rice (½ cup)—see recipe in Appendix A
Carrots (½ cup sprinkled with mint)

Metabo-Meal:

Fruit Mix with Yogurt Topping:
    Cantaloupe (½ cup diced)
    Honeydew (½ cup diced)
    Yogurt (¼ cup, plain, low-fat)

T U E S D A Y

Breakfast:

Low-cal breakfast as prescribed

Lunch:

Vegetable Plate—see recipe in Appendix A

Dinner:

Fish Creole or Fish with Dill Sauce (5 ounces)—see recipes in
    Appendix A

Baked potato (½ baked)
Mixed vegetables (½ cup mix of any two vegetables; for
example, carrots and cauliflower)

Metabo-Meal:

Pear or apple (1 whole)

W E D N E S D A Y

Breakfast:

Low-cal breakfast as prescribed

Lunch:

Macaroni Salad (1½ cups)—see recipe in Appendix A

Dinner:

Italian Chicken or Chicken Parmesan (1 breast)—see recipe in
Appendix A
Wild rice (½ cup)
Broccoli (½ cup)

Metabo-Meal:

Cereal (¾ cup of any prescribed breakfast cereal)
Milk (½ cup of skim or 2 percent low-fat)

T H U R S D A Y

Breakfast:

Low-cal breakfast as prescribed

Lunch:

Pita Sandwich:
Pita bread (1) stuffed with:
    Tuna (½ ounce of water-packed with 1 teaspoon diet
      margarine)
    Tomato (½ cup, chopped)
    Lettuce (1 cup, chopped)
    Onion (1 tablespoon, chopped)

Dinner:

Spaghetti (1 cup of cooked noodles)
Tomato sauce (¼ cup commercially prepared or ½ cup if recipe
    in Appendix A is used)
Parmesan cheese (1 teaspoon sprinkled on top)
Italian bread (1 piece with 1 teaspoon diet margarine)

Metabo-Meal:

Fruit Ambrosia—see recipe in Appendix A

F R I D A Y

Breakfast:

Low-cal breakfast as prescribed

Lunch:

Cantaloupe (½), topped with:
    Cottage cheese (¼ cup, low fat)
    Strawberries (½ cup, sliced)
Crackers or melba toast (3)

Dinner:

Veal Piccata (3 ounces)—see recipe in Appendix A
Egg noodles (½ cup)
Zucchini (½ cup)

Metabo-Meal:

Banana (1 whole, medium)

S A T U R D A Y   A N D   S U N D A Y

• *Refer to the next chapter for Booster Weekend Menu Plans.*

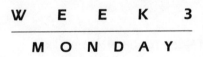

W E E K   3

M O N D A Y

Breakfast:

Low-cal breakfast as prescribed

Lunch:

Stuffed Baked Potato (1 medium)
    Stuffed with:
    Low-cal Cheddar cheese (½ slice, melted in potato)

Broccoli (4 ounces, cooked)
Dessert:
  Banana (¼ sliced)
  Yogurt (1 tablespoon plain)

Dinner:

Chicken Enchilada with Salsa—see recipe in Appendix A
Brown rice (¼ cup)

Metabo-meal:

Seedless grapes (½ cup)

T U E S D A Y

Breakfast:

Low-cal breakfast as prescribed

Lunch:

Crabmeat Salad—see recipe in Appendix A

Dinner:

Baked fish (5 ounces—any fish, prepared according to any of
    the fish recipes in Appendix A)
Roasted Chips (½ potato)—see recipe in Appendix A
Spinach (½ cup)

Metabo-Meal:

Cereal (¾ cup of any prescribed breakfast cereal)
Milk (½ cup skim or 2 percent low-fat)

W E D N E S D A Y

Breakfast:

Low-cal breakfast as prescribed

Lunch:

Chicken or Turkey Sandwich:
    Chicken or Turkey (1-ounce slice)
    Low-cal mayonnaise (1 teaspoon)
    Tomato (2 slices)
    Lettuce (1 medium leaf)

Dinner:

Baked Ziti (1 cup)—see recipe in Appendix A
Small tossed salad (with 1 tablespoon diet salad dressing)

Metabo-Meal:

Popcorn (4 cups, air-popped, no butter or salt)

T H U R S D A Y

Breakfast:

Low-cal breakfast as prescribed

Lunch:

Large Tossed Salad:
    Lettuce (2 cups of iceberg, Bibb, or romaine)
    Tomato (1, sliced or diced)
    Onion rings (3)
    Green pepper rings (2)
    Celery (1 stalk, diced)
    Low-cal salad dressing (3 tablespoons)
Melba toast or crackers (4)

Dinner:

Lamb with Mint Sauce (2 small chops)—see recipe in
    Appendix A
Mashed Potato (1 medium)—see recipe in Appendix A
Peas/carrot mix (½ cup peas mixed with ¼ cup diced carrots)

Metabo-Meal:

Grapefruit (1 whole), topped with:
    Cinnamon (1 teaspoon)
    Artificial sweetener (1 packet)

F R I D A Y

Breakfast:

Low-cal breakfast as prescribed

Lunch:

Pita Pizza—see recipe in Appendix A

Dinner:

Shrimp Curry or Shrimp Scampi (5 ounces)—see recipe in Appendix A

Metabo-Meal:

Choose any one of your favorite Low-Cal Menu Metabo-Meals

Substitutions and Variations

The closer you stick to my menu plan the more successful you will be. For variety, however, you may use the main-dish recipes in Appendix A as substitutes for any main dishes that don't appeal to you or that contain foods to which you are allergic. Just make sure that you substitute a recipe in the same food category; for example, chicken for chicken, pasta for pasta, etc.

Because fruits are seasonal, feel free to substitute any of the following fruit portions for one another:

Apple (1 whole)
Banana (1 whole)
Grapefruit (1 whole)
Orange (1 whole)
Pear (1 whole)
Strawberries (¾ cup)
Grapes (¾ cup)
Cantaloupe (¼)
Honeydew (⅛)
Watermelon (1 cup, diced)
Peach (1 whole)
Plums (2 whole)
Raisins (1½ tablespoons)

Most vegetables can be substituted freely as long as the portion size is the same. The only exceptions are peas, corn, parsnips, and lima beans. You should use half the recommended portion size when substituting these vegetables for any other in the menu plan.

If you have food allergies, simply substitute foods in the same nutritional category. For example, substitute protein for protein, carbohydrate for carbohydrate, etc. If you have extensive food allergies I would suggest you consult your physician or a nutritionist to help you make appropriate substitutions to suit your particular allergy.

Now let's look at what you should eat during the Booster Weekends.

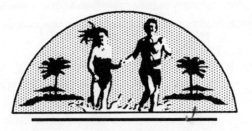

C H A P T E R 8

The Booster Weekend Menu Plan

On every Saturday and Sunday you should follow my Booster Weekend Menu Plan. You will notice that this plan requires you to eat slightly more calories at each meal and also provides you with a second Metabo-Meal. *It is essential that you switch from the Low-Cal Menu Plan to this Booster Menu Plan on weekends.*

I am providing you with menu plans for three weekends. If reaching your ideal weight takes longer, simply repeat the three-weekend sequence once again.

Weekend 1

S A T U R D A Y

Breakfast

Cereal (¾ cup Raisin Bran, All-Bran, or Mueslix; make certain you
choose one of these high-fiber cereals)
Milk (½ cup skim or 2 percent low-fat)
Fruit (1 whole; choice of orange or banana)

Lunch

Hamburger:
    Lean Hamburger (3 ounces)
    Hamburger bun (1 whole-wheat)

Metabo-Meal:

Fruit (1 whole; choice of apple or pear)

Dinner:

Macaroni and Cheese, Vermicelli Sciacca, or Fettuccine
    Alfredo (1 cup of your choice)—see recipes in Appendix A ᵖG. 16
Small tossed salad (with 2 tablespoons of diet salad dressing)
Italian bread (1 piece; no butter or margarine)

Metabo-Meal:

Cereal (¾ cup of any Low-Cal or Booster cereal)
Milk (½ cup skim or 2 percent low-fat)

S U N D A Y

Breakfast:
Choice of either:

Egg (1 poached, hard boiled, or fried in low-calorie
vegetable cooking spray)
Bread (2 slices of diet, whole-wheat)
Jelly (2 tablespoons; diet-type)
Orange (1 whole)

or

French Toast (3 slices)—see recipe in Appendix A
Syrup (1 tablespoon; diet type)
Orange (1 whole)

Lunch:

Watermelon (1 pound)
Cantaloupe (¼, diced)
Strawberries (½ cup, sliced)
Cottage cheese (⅔ cup, low-fat)
Melba toast (4)

Metabo-Meal:

Fruit (1 apple, orange, banana, or pear)

Dinner:

Filet mignon (4 ounces steak)
Mashed Potatoes (⅔ cup)—see recipe in Appendix A
Mixed vegetables (1 cup; carrots, onions, peas)

Metabo-Meal:

Popcorn (4 cups of air-popped; no butter or salt)

Weekend 2

S A T U R D A Y

Breakfast:

Same as Weekend 1 Saturday breakfast

Lunch:

Egg Salad Sandwich:
Egg (1 whole hard-boiled; chopped with 1 teaspoon low-cal
mayonnaise added)
Tomato (2 slices)
Lettuce (1 leaf)
Bread (2 slices; diet whole-wheat)
Soup (1 cup low-sodium vegetable, either purchased or made
from recipe in Appendix A)

Metabo-Meal:

Banana/Strawberry Surprise:
Banana (½ medium, sliced)
Strawberries (½ cup, sliced)
Yogurt (1 tablespoon low-fat, plain, used as a topping for
the fruit mixture)

Dinner:

Baked fish (5 ounces)—use any recipe in Appendix A

Rice (½ cup with 1 teaspoon diet margarine)
Broccoli (½ cup)
Tossed salad (small bowl with 1 teaspoon diet dressing)

Metabo-Meal:

Cereal (¾ cup of any Booster Saturday breakfast cereal)
Milk (½ cup skim or 2 percent low-fat)

S U N D A Y

Breakfast:

Same choice as Weekend 1 Sunday breakfast

Lunch:

Turkey Sandwich:
    Turkey (3 ounces, sliced turkey)
    Mayonnaise (1 tablespoon, low-calorie)
    Tomato (2 slices)
    Lettuce (1 medium leaf)
    Bread (2 slices, diet whole-wheat)

Metabo-Meal:

Fruit (1 whole apple, banana, peach, pear, orange)

Dinner:

Pasta and Veggies (1 cup)—see recipe in Appendix A

Metabo-Meal:

Cereal (¾ cup of any prescribed breakfast cereal)
Milk (½ cup skim or 2 percent low-fat)

Weekend 3

S A T U R D A Y

Breakfast:

Same as Saturday breakfast for Booster Weekend 1

Lunch:

Egg-White Omelet (2 portions)—see recipe in Appendix A

Metabo-Meal:

Raw Vegetable Plate:
    Carrots (6 medium sticks)
    Celery (6 medium sticks)
    Radishes (3 whole)
    Cauliflower (½ cup florets)

Dinner:

Cheese Manicotti (1 portion)—see recipe in Appendix A
Italian bread (2 pieces with 1 teaspoon diet margarine)

Metabo-Meal:

Fruit Ambrosia—see recipe in Appendix A

S U N D A Y

Breakfast:

Same choice as Weekend 1 Sunday breakfast

Lunch:

Shrimp and Macaroni Salad (1½ cups)—see recipe in
Appendix A

Metabo-Meal:

Cereal (¾ cup of any prescribed Booster Saturday breakfast
cereal)
Milk (½ cup skim or 2 percent low-fat)

Dinner:

Chicken à la King (1 portion)—see recipe in Appendix A
Curried Rice (½ cup)—see recipe in Appendix A

Metabo-Meal:

Baked Apple (1 whole)—see recipe in Appendix A

If you choose to stay on the Hilton Head Over-35 Diet
longer, simply repeat these Booster Weekend Menus in the
same sequence. Once you reach your target weight, refer to
Chapter 13, which will tell you how to prepare your metabolism for maintenance calories.

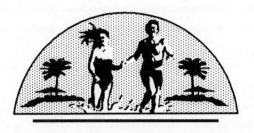

CHAPTER 9

Questions and Answers About My Low-Cal Weekday and Booster Weekend Menu Plans

Q. I have heard that I can slow down the aging process by taking megadoses of vitamin A, vitamin E, and the minerals selenium and zinc. Why don't you recommend these supplements?

A. As you know, I recommend a multivitamin/mineral supplement while you are dieting. Once you are eating a maintenance level of calories I, as well as most experts, believe that by eating a balanced diet you will get all of the vitamins and minerals you need from the foods you eat. While there are many theories suggesting that large doses of certain vitamins and minerals will slow down the aging process, there is absolutely no sound, scientific evidence that this is true. In fact, continued megadoses of vitamin A and selenium can be toxic.

Q. How much liquid should I drink on your diet?

A. You should drink at least four eight-ounce glasses of non-caffeinated beverages per day. I suggest water or noncaffeinated diet drinks. To keep your energy level high you must replace the fluid your body naturally loses through dieting and exercise. Since you are on a low-sodium diet you don't have to worry about retaining the fluids you are drinking. They will be flushed out of your system.

Q. I have heard that diet soft drinks and club soda have a lot of sodium. Should I restrict their usage if I have high blood pressure or if I am retaining too much fluid?

A. Diet soft drinks and club soda have about 35 milligrams of sodium per glass. Actually, this is not a great deal of sodium considering the fact that you are allowed as much as 2,000 milligrams of sodium per day for good health. Even so, I would suggest you limit yourself to no more than four glasses per day.

Q. I don't eat red meat of any kind. I notice that your menus call for veal, lamb, steak, or roast beef about once a week. What can I substitute?

A. It is perfectly okay for you to substitute any of the fish or poultry dinners for the red meat dinners I prescribe. Many people prefer not to eat red meat in an attempt to cut down on cholesterol. Most doctors agree, however, that red meat once a week is perfectly acceptable for treating a high cholesterol level. In fact, many would allow it twice each week.

Q. My husband and I both have high blood pressure. Is it safe for us to go on the Hilton Head Over-35 Diet?

A. In addition to helping you lose weight, the Hilton Head Over-35 Diet may also help to control your blood pressure. Many clients who have lost weight at the Institute have been able to reduce or eliminate their blood-pressure medication. This is a healthy diet designed not only for the metabolic problems of the over-35 group but their medical problems as well. However, because you have high blood pressure you should consult your physician before you begin this or any diet. He or she may want to monitor your blood pressure throughout the diet and may have to lower your medication accordingly. Never reduce your blood-pressure medication on your own without your physician's advice.

Q. If I am planning to eat in a restaurant for lunch or dinner, can I substitute a meal from another day if that will make it easier for me to order?

A. I would suggest that you first try to order what my menu plan calls for on that particular day. If this is not possible, you may switch as long as the meals consist of approximately the same types of nutrients. For example, you may substitute a fish for a chicken meal or vice versa but you should not substitute a fish meal (protein) for a pasta meal (complex carbohydrate).

Q. If I will be going to a dinner party or a restaurant on the weekend, can I skip my afternoon or evening Metabo-Meal and use the extra calories for dinner?

A. Absolutely not. Once you start doing this, you begin to change the system and it will no longer work as well for you. Five meals on weekends are essential in order to properly stimulate your metabolism.

Q. My body seems to require more protein than the Hilton Head Over-35 Diet calls for. In fact, I lose weight faster on high-protein diets. Can I modify your diet to include more protein?

A. No. Not under any circumstances. The only reason some people lose weight a little faster in the beginning of a high-protein diet is that they are losing more water. This is an artificial water loss that will be regained as soon as the diet is stopped. And, as I have said previously, high protein diets rob your body of muscle tissue, causing even more damage to your metabolism. The high proportion of complex carbohydrates in the Hilton Head Over-35 Diet will ensure that you save your muscle and burn the fat instead.

Q. What if I lose control of my appetite one day and overeat? Should I eat less the next day to compensate?

A. Definitely not. The best thing to do is simply go right back on the menu plans as I have outlined them. One eating episode usually only puts on water weight, not fat weight. Forgive yourself and act like your mistake never happened. In a later chapter I will be giving you the secrets of my Hilton Head Motivational Plan, which will help you avoid such slip-ups.

Q. I am 60 years old and a diabetic. I take insulin every day. My doctor has advised me to lose 30 pounds. Is your diet safe for diabetics?

A. Yes, it is. We often treat diabetics at the Hilton Head Health Institute and they do very well on the diet. They not only lose weight but some have been able to reduce their dependence on insulin. One of our clients, who happened to be a physician, monitored his blood-sugar level every day during his 26-day stay at our Institute. By the end of his stay he no longer required his daily insulin injection. Consult your physician first and ask his advice. I'm certain he or she will encourage you to begin the Hilton Head Over-35 Diet immediately, although probably with medical supervision.

Q. I am a 45-year-old woman with two teenage sons. My husband and I both want to lose 20 pounds. Can I put the whole family on your diet?

A. It certainly would be easier if you could. However, if your sons are younger than 18 I would not recommend my diet. Your boys would require more calories than most adult diets recommend. You could serve the same meals to everyone and give them larger portions and/or more items (such as an extra roll or piece of fruit).

Q. I find that foods without sauces, ketchup, mustard, etc., taste bland and unappealing. Can I use such toppings on your diet?

A. No, you may not. Sauces and condiments contain extra calories and usually a great deal of salt and sugar that you don't need. Actually, I want you to become accustomed to the taste of foods in their natural state. This is a key to long-term success. In addition, my recipes will provide dietary sauces that will spice up the meals. All of these recipes have been tested at the Hilton Head Health Institute and have won resounding praise from the participants in our programs.

Q. How much weight can I expect to lose on the Hilton Head Over-35 Diet?

A. This varies considerably, depending on the person. Women generally lose between 12 and 15 pounds during their 26-day stay at our Institute. Because of their stronger metabolic rates men lose between 16 and 20 pounds in 26 days.

Your weight loss may be higher or lower than these averages based on how much weight you have to lose or how sluggish your metabolism is. Just remember, how quickly you lose weight is not as important as losing those unwanted pounds *permanently*. If your body's metabolism does not respond as quickly as you would like, keep at it. If your body has undergone years of underactivity and fad dieting, it may take a little longer to stir up your metabolism. Don't get discouraged. Once we tune up your metabolic engine you'll be racing toward your ideal weight in no time at all.

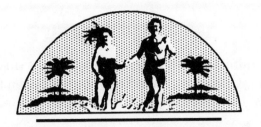

CHAPTER 10

Thermal Walking: The Best Fat Burner of All

The first thing I want you to know about my thermal-walking exercise plan is that it is easy and safe. All you have to do is walk at a moderate pace every day. Your thermal walks will be divided into two sessions with the total time for all of your exercise not exceeding 60 minutes on any day. My thermal-walking program is designed especially for people over 35 and does not require strenuous activity of any kind. If you can walk, even slowly, you will succeed with this program.

Before I go into detail about exactly how I want you to exercise, let's quickly look at why you should exercise in the first place. Regular physical activity is essential for the over-35 body because it:

1. *Burns Fat*—Whole-body-movement exercises such as walking, bicycling, and swimming are essential on a daily

basis in order to condition your aging metabolism and help it burn fat. Many studies have shown regular exercise is the most important key to long-term weight maintenance, especially as you get older.

2. *Strengthens Muscle*—Exercise also firms and strengthens muscle tissue which, as I have already explained, must be conditioned if you are to keep your metabolism strong with age. Since exercise like walking primarily strengthens leg muscles, you should include upper-body muscle-firming exercise routines as well.

3. *Prolongs Life*—Recent studies have proven that even moderate exercise, if scheduled on a regular basis, will add years to your life. Regular exercise can be especially beneficial to those with high blood pressure or with a family history of early death from stroke or heart disease. If you are in either of these categories, even moderate exercise can increase your lifespan dramatically. In a study of Harvard alumni (some of whom graduated over 60 years ago) those who walked as little as a mile a day had a 25 percent lower mortality rate than those who were inactive.

4. *Strengthens Bones*—Regular exercise even makes your bones stronger by building up bone mineral mass. This is especially good news for women because exercise can help prevent the thinning of the bones that occurs with age. These bone changes, known as osteoporosis, increase your risk of bone fracture and compression of the spine. While the calcium supplementation I have recommended is necessary to help prevent this condition, exercise is also a crucial part of a total prevention program.

Why Thermal Walks Are the Best Exercise for Losing Weight

As you will recall from chapter 7, one of my Five Essential Rules of the Hilton Head Over-35 Diet is to exercise *after* meals every day. Because your metabolism increases for several hours after meals in order to adapt to the demands of digesting, absorbing, and transporting food, it is especially primed at that time to further enhancement.

Not only does exercise increase the normal metabolic boost you receive from meals but this thermogenesis also supercharges the effects of exercise. What this means is that you get more calorie burning out of exercise that occurs immediately after meals than exercise at any other time.

Keep in mind that:

AFTER-MEAL EXERCISE IS THE MOST EFFICIENT WAY TO LOSE WEIGHT

You could walk a mile during the afternoon and it simply wouldn't burn as many calories as a walk immediately after lunch. This is great news because now you can get more out of your exercise and burn more calories in less time.

The cornerstone of my exercise plan for you is known as the *thermal walk*. This is a walk immediately after a meal. *My program requires you to take two thermal walks a day.* I believe that of all the possible exercises you could choose from, walking after meals is the best for your over-35 body. Walking burns about the same number of calories as running and it results in fewer injuries to your back, knees, and muscles. The number of calories you burn while exercising is more related to *when* you exercise (for example, after a meal) and *how long* you exercise (for example, how many miles you walk) as opposed to the *intensity* of your exercise.

You simply don't need to exercise strenuously to lose weight effectively. Walking is the safest and surest way to rejuvenate your metabolism and firm your body. Unfortunately, I have seen too many people in their 40s and 50s begin a running or aerobic dance program in order to lose weight only to be stricken by muscle or joint injuries after only a few days. Then they can't exercise at all and gain even more weight.

Although I believe thermal walking to be your best weight-loss exercise, there are a few alternative exercises that I would approve. Bicycling (either outdoor or stationary), treadmill walking, and low-impact aerobics (during which you do not lose contact with the floor) are acceptable alternatives for a change of pace. Of course, these exercises must be performed *after* a meal. Swimming is okay occasionally but not as an exclusive thermal exercise (unless an injury or medical condition prevents you from walking). Recent evidence suggests that swimming may not be nearly as good as walking, especially if weight loss is your goal.

When to Do Your Thermal Walks

You should schedule two thermal walks a day, every day of the week. Regular walking, each and every day, is important if you are going to stimulate your metabolism. Your walks, one long and one short, should be scheduled as follows:

Thermal Walk 1

Your first thermal walk of the day should be right after breakfast. You may have to get up a little earlier in the morning to fit this in. *During this first exercise session of the day you should walk for 40 full minutes.* It is essential that you walk continuously with no stopping. This early morning thermal walk will stir up your metabolism and get it off to a good start for the day.

Thermal Walk 2

You can take your second thermal walk after any other meal during the day. It is best to take this walk after lunch or dinner, but you may occasionally take it after your Metabo-Meal if you choose. *This second thermal walk should last 20 minutes.*

How Fast and How Far You Should Walk

When you first begin the Hilton Head Metabolism Diet your pace of walking will depend on your overall fitness level and how much you weigh. If you haven't exercised on a daily basis, *it is vital that you start out very, very slowly.* I don't want you to injure yourself. Remember, you are beginning a lifetime of walking; you are not trying to make up for all your past years of inactivity in the next few weeks. Slow and steady, not sweat and strain, should be your motto.

Your goal should be to walk at a pace of one mile in 15 to 20 minutes. At this rate you could walk 2 to 2⅔ miles during Thermal Walk 1 and 1 to 1⅓ miles during Thermal Walk 2.

However, the first five minutes of each walk should be thought of as a warm-up phase during which you walk at a slightly slower pace. Start out with a leisurely stroll and gradually increase your pace during the first five minutes. Then level off to a pace of 15 to 20 minutes a mile for the rest of the walk.

How to Know If You Are Overdoing It

Based on my experiences at the Hilton Head Health Institute, I am more concerned about your pushing yourself too hard than not exercising strenuously enough. Most people who start a diet or fitness program want to go all-out from the very first day. This is especially true if you haven't exercised in a very long time or if, in the past, you were very active or athletic. Past athletes forget how the years have taken their toll and remember what they used to be able to do. At age 40, after years of inactivity, they feel they should be able to exercise the way they did at age 20. This approach usually results in sore muscles and injury to the back or the knees.

If you haven't been physically active in a long time (or ever), start out very slowly. You might even begin at a 30-minute-a-mile pace or more.

In addition to walking slowly for the first five minutes of your walk in order to limber up, you can take the *Perceived Exertion Test* during your walk to see if you are overdoing it. This test consists of a simple scale on which you rate how much effort you are putting into your walk. About halfway into your walk ask yourself, "How much effort is involved in the current pace of my walk?" Then rate your effort according to one of the following categories:

1. Very, very light
2. Very light
3. Fairly light
4. Somewhat hard
5. Hard
6. Very hard
7. Very, very hard

You should never exceed category 5 while walking. Most people who are walking within safe limits would rate their effort as category 3, 4, or 5. If you ever rate yourself in the "very hard" to "very, very hard" categories, *slow down immediately.* This indicates you are walking much too fast for your fitness level.

Although the Perceived Exertion Test is based on your opinion of how much effort you are exerting, it is actually more scientific than it appears. These ratings correspond very well to actual heart-rate measures and can serve as an accurate as well as simple indication of the safety of your walking pace.

One other simple measure of whether you are overdoing your exercise is called the *Talk Test.* Simply stated, if you can carry on a normal conversation while doing your thermal walks, you are probably exercising at a safe level. If you are out of breath and find it difficult to talk to someone while walking, you are going much too fast.

But remember—and this is important—if you are very overweight, have to lose over 50 pounds, or have an orthopedic or cardiac problem, consult your physician to establish the level of activity that's right for you.

Walking Shoes

The best thing about walking is that the only exercise equipment you need is a good pair of walking shoes. Nowadays with so much emphasis on fitness there are many shoes to choose from. I'm not just talking about a substantial pair of tennis shoes or a comfortable pair of flat "street" shoes. Walking or running shoes are constructed in a special way to protect you from injury. They have a well-cushioned heel and a very supportive arch.

Believe me, they are well worth the money in terms of

comfort and prevention of knee, ankle, and foot injuries. Even people with lower back pain and disk problems find that these shoes cushion the impact of their steps and protect them from back pain.

You can buy walking or running shoes (either will do) at most shoe and sporting-goods stores.

What About Thermal Walking in Bad Weather?

Many people ask me what to do about thermal walks when it's raining, cold, or too hot outside. My usual response is to tell them to walk in spite of the weather. I want you to get into a routine, and if you avoid your walk every time the weather is bad, you'll never lose weight. Just make sure to dress according to the weather conditions. And if you are walking in hot weather make certain you drink plenty of water both before and after your walk.

On days that are particularly stormy you might choose one of the indoor alternatives I mentioned earlier such as an exercycle or treadmill. Indoor cross-country skiing machines are also good for this purpose.

Your Doctor's Advice

Even though this is a moderate exercise program, I suggest that you consult your physician before starting it. He or she may want to examine you first or give you a treadmill electrocardiogram (stress test). This is especially important if you are very overweight or have any significant risk factors such as the ones I listed on page 45.

I'm sure your physician will be pleased that you are going on such a well tested, sensible program. Physicians from all over the country refer patients to the Hilton Head Health Institute and have a great deal of confidence in our procedures. In fact, a great many physicians have participated personally in the program to overcome their own weight problems.

Are Thermal Walks All I Have to Do for Exercise?

While thermal walks are a fundamental part of the Hilton Head Over-35 Diet, they must be supplemented with exercises that increase muscle tissue. As you have learned, more muscle is an essential ingredient in stimulating your metabolism and making it young again. Thermal walks help you most by burning calories at a high rate and firming muscles in your legs and buttocks. They do little, however, for the muscles in the upper part of your body. Since we must increase muscle mass throughout your body, you must also use my upper-body Muscle Reconditioners. As you will see, these exercises need only be done three times a week and, because they take the place of Thermal Walk 2 on those days, they do not add any time to your total exercise program. You never have to exercise more than a total of one hour each day.

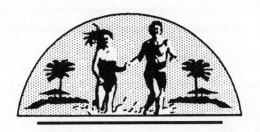

CHAPTER 11

Muscle Reconditioning for a Stronger Metabolism

In order to increase muscle tissue you will need exercises that place a real physical demand on your muscles. Muscle tissue is not increased simply by body movements such as walking, but requires what is known as *resistance training*. The muscle must work against a resistance such as a weight in order to get stronger and firmer. Even if you are quite physically active, unless you have a specific amount of resistance training, you will not be strengthening your muscle mass as much as is required for a youthful metabolism.

I have designed a simple yet effective method to help you increase muscle mass without having to become a professional weight lifter in the process. The goal is not to develop big, bulky muscles but, rather, strong, firm ones. (Because of your age, unless you started lifting weights early in life, you would have difficulty building big muscles even if you wanted to.) My muscle-reconditioning exercises will develop and strengthen the muscle fiber you already have and prevent further muscle loss.

The Case of the Muscle Resistance Resister

Occasionally I run into people in my program at the Hilton Head Health Institute who find the notion of muscle building difficult to accept. Anne, a 48-year-old interior designer from New York, is a classic example. When she first came to the Institute she weighed 154 pounds. At her height of 5-foot-6 and her small-to-medium body-frame size, we determined her ideal weight to be approximately 130 pounds. Her lean body mass percentage was only 64 percent, 11 percentage points lower than it should have been to keep her metabolism tuned up. She was greatly in need not only of fat loss but also muscle reconditioning. While she readily followed our dietary plan and took her scheduled thermal walks, she resisted the idea of muscle-firming exercises. Apparently the staff of a commercial weight-loss program in her community had convinced her that since muscle weighs more than fat, muscle exercises during a diet would slow down her weight loss. They even had her on a liquid-protein formula, and the combination of this low-carbohydrate diet and no exercise had devastating effects on her metabolism. Even so, she continued to believe that muscle exercises were bad for her.

While it is true that muscle weighs more than fat, muscle-reconditioning exercises will not slow your fat loss during a diet. In fact, what we find at the Institute is that since our participants are firming muscles as well as losing fat, they always look as if they lost more weight than they actually have. This is why we use body measurements, fat percentages, and lean-body-mass percentages as measures of progress along with weighing. As I mentioned previously, your weight on the scale is only one indication of how you are doing.

By not doing muscle-reconditioning exercises, you will hold your metabolism back and you won't be able to burn as many calories or fully stimulate and rejuvenate your aging metabolism.

I finally convinced Anne of these facts and she began our muscle reconditioning program. In four weeks she lost 16 pounds and looked firm and trim. Her body responded well to the muscle reconditioners. She put it this way:

> I love the feeling of strength and firmness I get from your muscle reconditioners. And you were right. The exercises didn't keep me from losing weight. I feel as if my body and metabolism are coming alive again. I'm starting to look and feel years younger.

When Anne returned home to New York after her program at the Institute was over she continued to lose weight. It took her three more weeks to get down to her goal of 130 pounds. She continues to do her thermal walks and muscle reconditioners.

In fact, when she first arrived home with her 16-pound weight loss, her husband and friends swore that she looked as if she had lost over 20 pounds. Actually, they were responding to the results of the muscle reconditioning program. Anne lost her fat, firmed and strengthened her muscle, and looked absolutely fantastic!

When and How Often

You should schedule my eight muscle reconditioners three times a week. They shouldn't take more than 20 minutes to perform. To keep your program simple and less time consuming I suggest you substitute your muscle-reconditioning routine for Thermal Walk 2 on either Monday, Wednesday, and Friday or Tuesday, Thursday, and Saturday. You must have a day of rest between your muscle-reconditioning exercises so schedule them on alternating days of the week.

You should perform the muscle reconditioners a maximum of three times a week. Your muscles will respond best with this schedule and you will not accomplish more by scheduling more frequent sessions.

Equipment You Will Need

For the muscle reconditioners, all you need is a pair of hand-held weights. You don't need the big "dumbbell" weights that weight lifters use. Go to your local discount or sporting-goods store and you will find a variety of hand-held weights. Any style will do. You can purchase the simple black iron ones or the chrome- or plastic-coated ones. Appearance really doesn't matter, so the choice is completely up to you and your budget.

Choose a weight that is light enough for you to lift with one arm about ten times without becoming overly fatigued. Women usually start out by using three- to five-pound weights while men can often handle six to eight pounds. As you become stronger and firmer you might want to slowly increase the size of the weights you are using. Just keep in mind that if you have to strain to complete these exercises you are using too much weight.

Some Important Precautions

You should always consult your physician before embarking on this or any other exercise program. He may want to evaluate your medical fitness before you begin in addition to supervising your progress.

To avoid injury make certain to complete the muscle reconditioners exactly as I have outlined them. These exercises have been designed to protect your over-35 body, especially your lower back and joints. You may already have problems in these areas and we certainly don't want to aggravate them.

It is essential to do these exercises in a smooth, easy motion. Don't rush them or try to do more than I prescribe. Don't use weights that are so heavy that you have to sweat and strain to complete the movements. At the Institute a number of people, because of their age and poor fitness level, started out doing these muscle reconditioners with no weights at all.

Make sure to breathe normally while you are doing the muscle reconditioners. You may have a tendency to hold your breath as you lift the weights, but you must regularly monitor your breathing and be sure not to hold your breath. It is definitely not good practice for anyone and could be particularly dangerous if you suffer from high blood pressure.

Eight Muscle Reconditioners

To firm muscle tissue and increase your metabolism, complete these exercises three times each week. The descriptions and the drawings will show you exactly what to do.

Muscle Reconditioner 1: Arm Curls

- Stand straight with arms at your sides, holding one weight in each hand. Palms should be facing forward.
- Bending your right arm at the elbow, lift the weight up to your shoulder. Then slowly bring it back down.
- Repeat 12 to 15 times. Rest for a few seconds and do 12

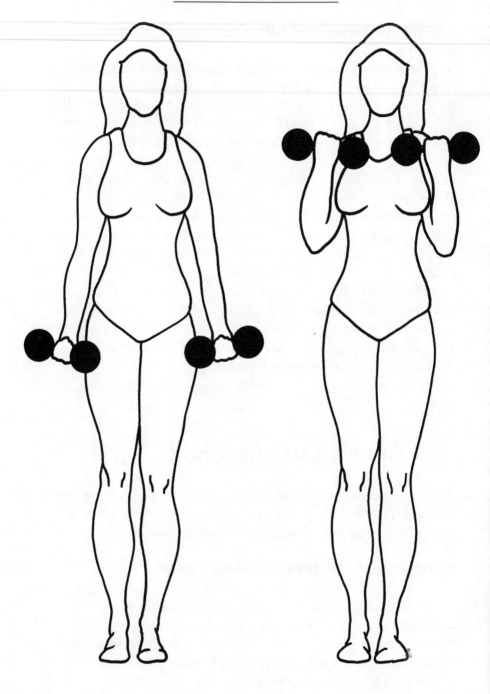

to 15 more repetitions with the same arm. Now repeat with the left arm.

• If you are unable to lift the weight 12 to 15 times, the weights you are using are too heavy for you.

Muscle Reconditioner 2: Arm Lifts

• Stand straight with one weight in each hand. Lift your arms out straight to your sides palms up, all the way up to shoulder level, so that your arms are parallel to the floor. Keep your arms straight, but do not lock your elbows.

• Slowly bring your arms back down to your sides. Repeat slowly 12 to 15 times. Rest for a few seconds and do 12 to 15 more repetitions.

Muscle Reconditioner 3: Side Bends

• With your arm bent, elbow pointing to the side, hold one weight on your shoulder. The other arm should be straight down at your side with the weight in your hand.

• Bend sideways toward your straight-arm side until you feel the muscles along the other side of your body stretching out. Straighten, repeat 12 to 15 times, rest, and repeat once more.

• Switch arm positions and repeat two sets of 12 to 15 repetitions each on the other side.

Muscle Reconditioner 4: Military Press

• With your arms bent, elbows pointing to the front, hold the weights on your shoulders. Push both weights straight up until your arms are perfectly straight over your head.

• Bring the weights down to your shoulders in a slow, fluid motion. Repeat 12 to 15 times, rest and repeat 12 to 15 more times.

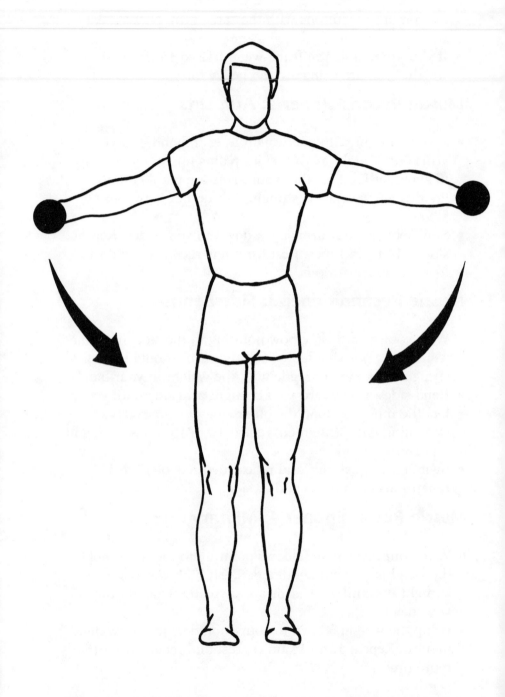

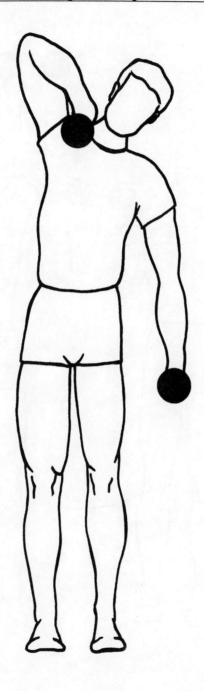

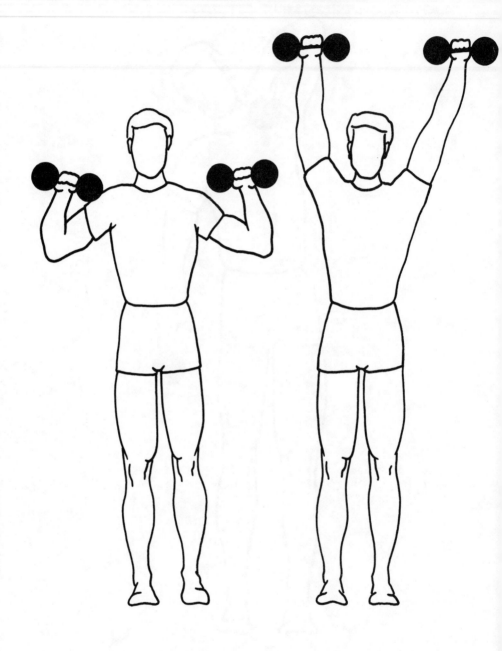

Muscle Reconditioner 5: Triceps Extension

- Hold only one weight. Start with your arms straight down, palms facing outward. Raise your hand and arm with the weight straight up from your shoulder and over your head.
- Bending your arm at the elbow, let the weight fall slowly backward toward the upper part of your back. With your other hand, brace your elbow near your head, to keep the elbow from moving.
- Lift the weight back up, so your arm is fully extended over your head again. Let the weight fall backward and grip your bent elbow. Keep your elbow steady and facing forward.
- Repeat 12 to 15 times, rest, and repeat 12 to 15 times again. Switch the weight to the other hand and repeat.

Muscle Reconditioner 6: Straight-Arm Lifts

- Lie on your back with your knees bent and your arms perpendicular to your body. Hold the weights in your hands, palms facing upward.
- Bend your arms slightly at the elbows, and smoothly lift the weights above your body so that your hands come in contact with one another. Keep your lower back pressed to the floor.
- Slowly bring your arms back down to the floor. Do 12 to 15 repetitions two times.
- Keep your knees bent as you do this exercise. This presses your lower back to the floor, strengthening your stomach muscles.

Muscle Reconditioner 7: Bench Press

- Lie flat on your back on the floor, knees bent, arms perpendicular to your body, holding a weight in each

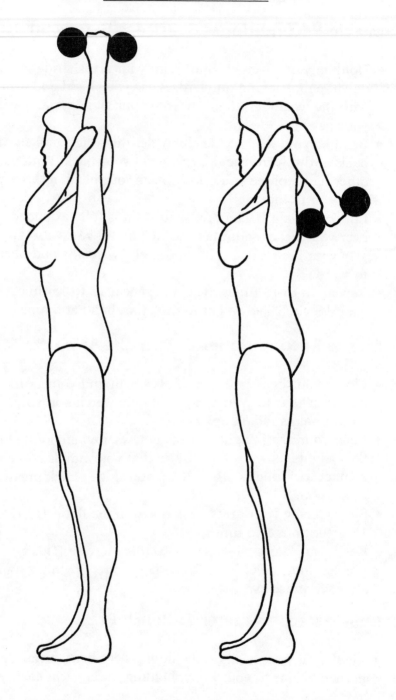

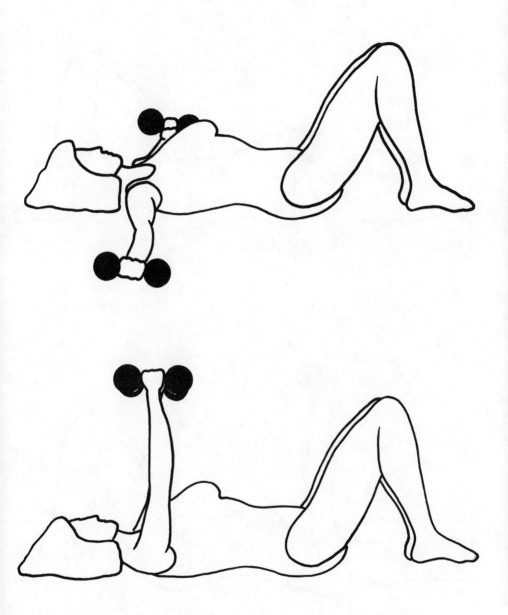

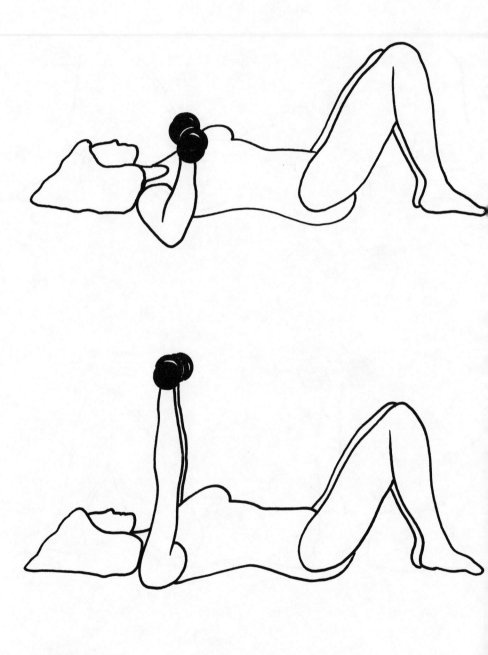

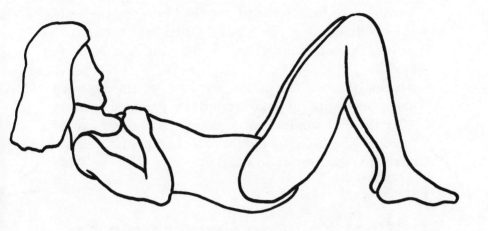

hand. Bend your elbows so that they rest on the floor by your sides and you are holding the weights up in the air. Your palms should be facing outward toward your toes.

- Push both arms up simultaneously so that your arms are straight and fully extended upward. Do not allow your lower back to arch off the floor during this extension.
- Slowly bring your arms down, resting your elbows on the floor once again. Repeat 12 to 15 times, in a slow, fluid motion. Rest and repeat 12 to 15 more times.

Muscle Reconditioner 8: Abdominal Curls

You will not need your hand weights for this exercise.

- Lie on your back with your knees bent and your feet flat on the floor. Fold your hands across your chest. *Never do this exercise with your legs straight. Your legs must be bent to protect your lower back from strain.*

- Curl your body up slowly to a 30-degree angle, starting by moving your head forward and then bringing the rest of your body up, *very, very* slowly. Come back down just as slowly. Do not sit up all the way but only to a 30-degree angle.
- Repeat 10 times, rest and repeat 10 more times. Over a few weeks work up to 20 repetitions, repeated 3 times. After these abdominal curls become easier, you can increase resistance by holding a 2- to 3-pound weight against your chest as you curl up.

What You Can Expect from the Muscle Reconditioners

While our major purpose for the eight muscle-reconditioning exercises is to increase lean body mass and, thus, rejuvenate your metabolism, you will notice a number of other benefits as well. You will be stronger and have more energy and stamina. You will feel that strength in your body even when you are sitting or standing still.

Best of all, your body will begin to take on that young, firm appearance. Women especially notice differences in their waist and abdomen. You'll also notice your arms getting firmer, especially in the triceps area, on the back of your arm between your shoulder and elbow.

You'll find these muscle reconditioners easy and enjoyable. Before you know it your entire body will be shedding those excess pounds.

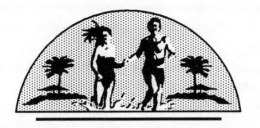

CHAPTER 12

Questions and Answers About Thermal Walking and Muscle Reconditioning

Q. I am a very busy person with very little time for exercise. Couldn't I accomplish just as much by taking thermal walks three times a week?

A. Definitely not. Thermal walking is one of the most important ingredients of the Hilton Head Over-35 Diet and it must be scheduled every day. While I realize that there may be an *occasional* day when you will not be able to take a thermal walk, exercising three times a week is not enough to stimulate your metabolism. I realize that many people lead busy lives with many responsibilities. However, if you want to keep your metabolism young and control your weight you *must* find the time for daily thermal walks.

Q. I have read that aerobic exercise three to four times a week is all that I need to keep my heart and lungs in shape. Why does your program require more exercise than this?

A. Don't confuse metabolic fitness with cardiovascular fitness. As you age, your metabolism requires daily thermal walks to keep it strong. Interestingly enough, your cardiovascular system doesn't need exercise as frequently as this for fitness.

Q. I must leave for work at 6:45 A.M. each morning since I have an hour commute to get there. How can I possibly do Thermal Walk 1 after breakfast? I would have to wake up before 5:30 A.M.

A. Unless you are an early-morning person I realize that such a schedule of thermal walking would be extremely difficult to maintain. Although I believe that thermal walking first thing in the morning is the optimum method of stimulating metabolism, I suggest you try to schedule your 40-minute thermal walk after lunch. If this is not possible, take your 20-minute thermal walk after lunch and do your longer walk after dinner. Depending on weather and darkness you may have to purchase an indoor treadmill or exercycle for this purpose.

Q. What if something comes up and I can't do my thermal walk for 20 or 30 minutes after I eat? Should I still walk or must I wait and walk after my next meal?

A. The thermogenic effect of a meal continues to stimulate your metabolism for two to three hours after your meal is eaten. While I feel it is better for you to walk right after you eat, the walk will still energize your metabolic rate even if you take it 20 or 30 minutes later.

Q. I am a 45-year-old man with most of my extra weight

in my stomach. Will your muscle reconditioners help me burn this fat faster?

A. Unfortunately, no matter what you've heard in the past, there is no such thing as spot reducing. When you diet and walk you lose fat all over your body as well as from your stomach. Muscle Reconditioner 8 (Abdominal Curls) will firm the muscles in your stomach and give it a firmer appearance, but you can only lose the fat through diet and thermal walks.

Q. Will your exercise program get rid of the cellulite in my hips and thighs?

A. Many people believe that cellulite is a special kind of dimply fat that women get on their hips, thighs, and buttocks. Actually, cellulite is normal, everyday fat. There is nothing special about it and no special pills, creams, or machines will get rid of it. The fat on your thighs and hips will be burned off when you diet and walk. It may be, however, that you have a hereditary predisposition to have more fat in the lower half of your body than in the upper half. While my muscle reconditioners will help firm your thighs and hips, you are not going to be able to totally resculpture your figure without the aid of plastic surgery.

Q. I have a slipped disk and suffer from lower back pain. Are your thermal walks and muscle reconditioners safe for me?

A. All of my exercises were developed with safety in mind. The muscle reconditioners will strengthen your muscles without hurting your back. However, you should check with your physician before starting this or any exercise program. He may want to modify the program based on your particular back problem. Many orthopedic specialists nowadays are encouraging their patients to stay active and avoid lengthy periods of bedrest that often weaken muscles that support the back.

Q. What if I have the flu for a few days and miss my thermal walks? When I recover should I double up on my exercise and try to do three or four thermal walks a day?

A. No. Just get back to your routine of two thermal walks a day. This all-or-nothing approach is a bad habit to start because you'll overexert yourself and possibly suffer an injury.

Q. On days when I have more time, is there anything wrong with extending my thermal walks for an extra 15 or 20 minutes?

A. Not at all. By all means, if you have the time and inclination, walk a little longer than I have prescribed. Just remember that I want you to get into a routine that you can continue for the rest of your life.

Q. In addition to stimulating my metabolism and keeping me trim and healthy, how else can thermal walks and muscle reconditioners help me?

A. Men and women who have followed my program of exercise report having more energy and stamina and a general sense of strength and well-being. Research has also shown that regular exercise of this nature improves your memory, creativity, and decision making. In addition, you will find that you experience fewer emotional ups and downs. Several people have even confided in me that because of my program their sex lives have never been better!

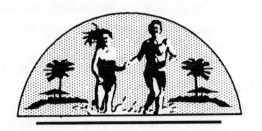

CHAPTER 13

What to Do When You Lose Your Weight: The Maintenance Ladder

Once you have lost all your excess weight you will be ready to climb the *maintenance ladder*. What I mean is that you should never go directly from a reducing diet to a maintenance diet overnight. Your metabolism is unable to handle such a quick change. In fact, unless you prepare your metabolism for the maintenance level of the program, you run the risk of gaining back two to three of the pounds you have just lost.

Getting Your Metabolism Accustomed to More Food

During the Hilton Head Over-35 Diet your metabolism has been burning very efficiently. Because food stimulates your metabolism, as soon as you increase calories in order to maintain your weight, your metabolism will really be in high gear. The Hilton Head Over-35 Diet will have tuned your metabolic engine and once you reach maintenance, it's a bit like taking your new race car out on the track and putting it through its paces.

Because your engine has not been run at full throttle for quite a while, you must gradually increase its speed before you press all the way down on the accelerator.

This reentry phase is accomplished by what I like to call climbing the maintenance ladder. *The maintenance ladder represents a caloric level that is approximately halfway between the calories in the Hilton Head Over-35 Diet and those your body requires to maintain your weight.*

Obviously, you cannot continue on the Hilton Head Over-35 Diet once you have reached your ideal weight or you will continue to lose weight. And I'm sure you'll want to start eating a normal amount of food without gaining weight.

Constructing Your Maintenance Ladder

On the day that your scale says you have reached your ideal weight, prepare yourself to go on the Maintenance Ladder phase of the diet for one week. Although you may be tempted to charge right into maintenance once you have lost your weight, you must climb the maintenance ladder for one full week.

To determine how many calories you should eat while climbing this ladder, refer to chapter 6. As you will recall, in that chapter I asked you to calculate your resting metabolic rate and to determine your *total caloric expenditure*. Total caloric expenditure refers to the number of calories your body requires to maintain your ideal weight. This number is your maintenance level.

The maintenance level that you came up with was expressed in terms of a range indicating the lowest and the highest number of calories needed to maintain your weight. For example, your range might have been from 1,700 calories to 2,100 calories a day.

The following chart will tell you how many calories are in your maintenance ladder. In order to construct your maintenance ladder we will be using the *low* number in your total caloric expenditure range as a reference point.

I recently calculated these numbers for Marie, a 39-year-old pediatrician who had been battling a weight problem most of her life. Once she reached 35, her problem worsened to the point that she was 40 pounds overweight. She was chronically tired and depressed. To look at her you would have thought she was 49, not 39. With the help of the Hilton Head Over-35

HOW MANY CALORIES IN YOUR MAINTENANCE LADDER?

If the low number in your total calorie expenditure range is between:	The number of calories in your maintenance ladder is:
1,450–1,550	1,250
1,551–1,650	1,300
1,651–1,750	1,350
1,751–1,850	1,400
1,851–1,950	1,450
1,951–2,050	1,500
2,051–2,150	1,550
2,151–2,250	1,600
2,251–2,350	1,650
2,351–2,450	1,700
2,451–2,550	1,750
2,551–2,650	1,800

Diet she successfully lost her 40 pounds and is now a totally rejuvenated woman and a more effective professional.

Marie's total calorie expenditure range was 1,685 to 2,050. Using 1,685 as our reference number, the chart indicated that her maintenance ladder should be approximately 1,350 calories. This meant that for the first week after she had lost her forty pounds, Marie was advised to eat 1,350 calories a day. During this one-week maintenance ladder her metabolism was being tuned for lifetime maintenance.

Putting the Maintenance Ladder into Practice

Now that you know the number of calories in *your* maintenance ladder, start eating this number of calories for *one full week*. The only exception to this rule is that if, because of a need to lose a great many pounds, you have been on the Hilton Head Over-35 Diet for more than three months, stay on the maintenance ladder for two weeks.

Your week on the maintenance ladder should consist of a full seven days. There is no need to eat more calories on the weekend during this phase. *However, you should be eating five meals a day—breakfast, lunch, dinner, and two Metabo-Meals.*

A simple way to increase calories on the maintenance ladder is to follow the general meal plans for either the Low-Cal Weekdays or Booster Weekends that I have outlined, adding sufficient calories to attain your maintenance ladder level. Low-Cal Weekday menus consist of approximately 800 calories a day while Booster Weekend menus have 1,100 calories a day.

You can simply increase portion sizes, having larger portions of cereal, fruit, vegetables, potatoes, etc. Another method of increasing calories is to substitute nondiet products for diet ones. For example, diet bread has 40 calories a slice while nondiet bread has 80 to 100 calories a slice. You can add almost 100 calories in a day simply by making this switch. You can also add calories by having a piece of fruit as a dessert for dinner or adding a salad or roll to a dinner or lunch meal. Just make sure you distribute your extra calories throughout the day. Don't add all of your extra calories to the dinner meal. Your metabolism functions more efficiently when those calories are spread out.

Sample Maintenance Ladder Meal Plan

Although the number of calories in your maintenance ladder meal plan will depend on your individual total caloric expenditure range, I will provide a sample meal plan to further illustrate how to plan this phase of the diet. As an example, I will use the case of Marie, the overweight pediatrician mentioned above. Marie's maintenance ladder consisted of 1,350 calories. Here is how she adapted Week 1 of the Hilton Head Over-35 Diet menu plan (found in chapters 7 and 8) to convert it into her maintenance ladder menu plan. She simply had to add 550 calories per day to the 800-calorie Low-Cal Weekday menu plan to obtain her 1,350-calorie maintenance ladder plan. Since the Booster Weekend plan contains 1,100 calories a day, Marie only needed to add 250 additional calories to the Saturday and Sunday meal plans.

Breakfast Every Day:

Cereal (1 cup)—choice of Special K, Raisin Bran, Just Right, Product 19, Nutri-Grain, ProGrain, corn flakes, shredded wheat, oatmeal

Milk (⅔ cup)—low-fat (2 percent) or skim only

Toast (1 slice)—whole-wheat with 1 teaspoon margarine

Fruit (½ piece)—choice of orange, banana, grapefruit, peach, pear, apple (or ¼ medium cantaloupe or ⅛ medium honeydew)

Coffee or tea—sugar substitute and/or dash of low fat or skim milk may be added, if desired

**NOTE: *Breakfast calories were increased by 160 simply by increasing the cereal allocation to 1 cup, allowing ⅔ as opposed to ½ cup of milk, and adding a piece of toast with margarine.*

M O N D A Y

Breakfast:

Maintenance Ladder Breakfast as prescribed

Lunch:

Turkey Sandwich:
  Turkey (2 ounces)
  Low-cal mayonnaise (1 teaspoon)
  Tomato (2 slices)
  Lettuce (1 medium leaf)
  Whole-wheat bread (2 slices)—nondietetic

Fruit/Yogurt Mix (mix ½ cup strawberries with 2 ounces plain low-fat yogurt)

**NOTE: *Lunch calories were increased by 150 by allowing an additional ounce of turkey in the sandwich, by changing the bread from dietetic to nondietetic, and by increasing the amount of strawberries in the Fruit/Yogurt Mix by ¼ cup.*

Metabo-Meal:

Apple or pear (1 whole)

**NOTE: *By adding this Metabo-Meal to the Weekday Menu Plan, Marie was able to increase her daily intake by another 100 calories.*

Dinner:

Baked fish (6 ounces cooked with 1 tablespoon lemon juice/1 teaspoon diet margarine combination)
Roasted Chips (1 whole potato)—see recipe in Appendix A
Green beans (⅔ cup)
Dinner roll (1)—no margarine

**NOTE: *Dinner calories were increased by 140 by increasing the fish portion from 5 to 6 ounces, by allowing a whole potato rather than a half, and by adding a roll to the meal.*

Metabo-Meal:

Seedless grapes (½ cup)

T U E S D A Y

Breakfast:

Maintenance Ladder Breakfast as prescribed

Lunch:

Primavera Salad 2½ cups (Pasta/vegetable combination)—see recipe in Appendix A

**NOTE: *The calories in this lunch were increased by 150 simply by providing an additional cup of Primavera Salad.*

Metabo-Meal:

Banana or orange (1 whole)

**NOTE: *By adding this Metabo-Meal to the Weekday Menu Plan, Marie was able to increase her daily intake by another 100 calories.*

Dinner:

Pork Tenderloin (4 ounces)
Carrots (½ cup, diced)
New potatoes (4 medium-size)
Dinner salad (small tossed salad with 1 tablespoon diet dressing)

**NOTE: *140 calories were added to this dinner meal by increasing the pork portion from 3 to 4 ounces, adding one additional New potato, and adding a small tossed salad.*

Metabo-Meal:

Cereal (¾ cup Special K, corn flakes, or Product 19)
Milk (½ cup skim or low-fat)

W E D N E S D A Y

Breakfast:

Maintenance Ladder Breakfast as prescribed

Lunch:

Pita Sandwich:
   Pita bread (1)
   Tuna salad (2 ounces)—see recipe in Appendix A
   Tomato (½ cup, chopped)
   Onion (1 tablespoon, chopped)
   Lettuce (¾ cup, chopped)
Orange (1 whole)

NOTE: *An extra ounce of tuna salad and an orange were added to this meal to provide an extra 150 calories.*

Metabo-Meal:

Peach (1 whole) or **plums** (2 whole)

**NOTE: *By adding this Metabo-Meal to the Weekday Menu Plan, Marie was able to increase daily intake by another 100 calories.*

Dinner:

Choice of Jamaican Chicken, Mexican Chicken, or Chicken Cacciatore (1 breast)—see recipes in Appendix A
Rice (½ cup)

Broccoli (½ cup)
Dinner roll (1 whole with 1 teaspoon diet margarine)

**NOTE: *Dinner calories were increased by 140 by providing an additional ¼ cup of rice and by adding a dinner roll to the meal.*

Metabo-Meal:

Apple (1 medium to large)

T H U R S D A Y

Breakfast:

Maintenance Ladder Breakfast as prescribed

Lunch:

Spinach and Mushroom Omelet—see recipe in Appendix A
Whole-wheat bread (1 slice, nondietetic with 1 teaspoon diet margarine)
Cantaloupe (½)

**NOTE: *Lunch calories were increased by 150 by changing the bread from dietetic to nondietetic, adding diet margarine, and increasing the portion of cantaloupe from ¼ to ½.*

Metabo-Meal:

Apple, orange, banana, or pear (1 whole)

**NOTE: *By adding this Metabo-Meal to the Weekday Menu Plan, Marie was able to increase her daily intake by another 100 calories.*

Dinner:

Lasagna (1½ servings)—see recipe in Appendix A
Garden salad (small tossed salad with lettuce, tomato, radishes, and 1 tablespoon low-fat dressing)

**NOTE: *Calories were increased in this meal simply by increasing the lasagna portion from 1 to 1½.*

Metabo-Meal:

Popcorn (4 cups of air-popped; no butter or salt)

F R I D A Y

Breakfast:

Maintenance Ladder Breakfast as prescribed

Lunch:

Large Tossed Salad:
   Lettuce (2 cups of iceberg, Bibb, or romaine)
   Tomatoes (2, sliced or diced)
   Onion rings (3)
   Green pepper rings (2)
   Low-cal salad dressing (2 tablespoons)
Honeydew melon (¼)

**NOTE: *Lunch calories were increased by 150 calories by adding one extra tomato to the salad and providing a honeydew melon instead of a pear.*

Metabo-Meal:

Choice of any breakfast fruit (1 whole)

NOTE: *By adding this Metabo-Meal to the Weekday Menu Plan, Marie was able to increase her daily intake by another 100 calories.*

Dinner:

Boiled shrimp (5 ounces)
Cocktail sauce (2 tablespoons of commercial sauce)
Corn on the cob (1 large ear with 2 teaspoons diet margarine)
Hawaiian Cole Slaw (¾ cup)—see recipe in Appendix A
Biscuit (1 medium)

NOTE: *140 calories were added to the dinner meal by changing the medium ear of corn to a large ear and by adding a biscuit.*

Metabo-Meal:

Cereal (¾ cup of any of the prescribed breakfast cereals)
Milk (½ cup skim or 2 percent low-fat)

S A T U R D A Y

Breakfast:

Same as Booster Weekend breakfast for Saturday in chapter 8

Lunch:

Hamburger:
Lean hamburger (4 ounces)
Hamburger bun (1 whole-wheat)
Catsup (1½ tablespoons)

**NOTE: *The calories in this meal were increased by 150 by adding 2 ounces to the size of the hamburger and by allowing catsup.*

Metabo-Meal:

Fruit (1 whole; choice of apple or pear)

Dinner:

Macaroni and Cheese, Vermicelli Sciacca, or Fettuccine Alfredo (1½ cups of your choice)—see recipes in Appendix A
Small tossed salad (with 2 tablespoons diet dressing)
Italian bread (1 piece; no butter or margarine)

**NOTE: *This meal was increased by 100 calories by increasing the portion of the main course from 1 cup to 1½ cups.*

Metabo-Meal:

Cereal (¾ cup of any Low-Cal or Booster cereal)
Milk (½ cup of skim or 2 percent low-fat)

S   U   N   D   A   Y

Breakfast:

Same as Booster Weekend breakfast for Sunday in chapter 8

Lunch:

Watermelon (1 pound)
Cantaloupe (½, diced)
Strawberries (½ cup, sliced)
Cottage cheese (¾ cup, low-fat)
Melba toast (6)

**NOTE: *150 calories were added by increasing the cantaloupe from ¼ to ½, by increasing the cottage cheese portion from ⅔ to ¾ cup, and by adding 2 extra pieces of melba toast.*

Metabo-Meal:

Fruit (1 whole apple, orange, banana, or pear)

Dinner:

Filet mignon (5 ounces)
Mashed Potatoes (1 cup)—see recipe in Appendix A
Mixed vegetables (1 cup; carrots, onions, peas)

**NOTE: *Dinner calories were increased by 100 simply by increasing the steak allowance from 4 to 5 ounces and by increasing the mashed-potato portion from ⅔ cup to 1 cup.*

Metabo-Meal:

Popcorn (4 cups of air-popped; no butter or salt)

You can see how easy it is to construct your maintenance-ladder menu plan by making a few simple additions to the Low-Cal Weekday and Booster Weekend plans.

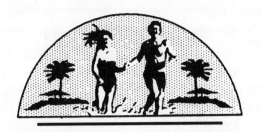

C H A P T E R 14

Five Lifetime Nutritional Guidelines

As you have learned, because of differences in age, body size, and gender, there is a tremendous variation in the number of calories people can eat at maintenance. However, Hilton Head Over-35 nutritional guidelines needed for maintenance of ideal weight are standard whether you are eating 1,200 calories or 3,200 calories.

The following are the Five Lifetime Maintenance Guidelines that you must put into practice in order to maintain your ideal weight. These guidelines will help you plan your meals and make food choices easier.

GUIDELINE 1: **Balance Your Nutrients by Eating 60 Percent Complex Carbohydrates, 15 Percent Protein, and No More Than 25 Percent Fat Each Day**

To keep your metabolism running strong and steady you must continue to feed it an abundance of complex carbohydrates in the form of fruit, vegetables, cereal, bread, pasta, and potatoes. Protein should comprise only 15 percent of your calories. Although your body's ability to digest and absorb protein declines with age, so does your overall need for protein. If you stick to my guidelines you will be eating as much protein as you require whether you are 40 or 80.

While 25 percent of your daily calories as fat may sound like a lot, it's really not much at all since fat is so calorically dense. That is, a little fat contains quite a few calories. For example, there are 100 calories in a tablespoon of oil. By not being careful you could easily add 400 or 500 calories to your daily intake just in the dressing poured on a salad.

Of the 25 percent of your calories coming from fat, no more than 10 percent of these should come from *saturated fats*. These are the "bad" fats that raise cholesterol. Saturated fats are found primarily in animal products such as red meat and organ meats such as liver, in butter, cheese, whole milk, cream, shortening, and egg yolks. Some vegetable oils such as palm oil and coconut oil are also bad for your cholesterol level since they contain even more saturated fat than butter!

Most of your fat intake should be in the form of either *polyunsaturated fats* or *monounsaturated fats*. Both of these fats actually help to lower your cholesterol so they are good for you. These good fats are found in the following oils:

Safflower
Corn
Sunflower
Soybean
Cottonseed
Olive
Peanut

The percentages of nutrients your body needs for maximum metabolic functioning should be based on the total number of calories you eat each day. Therefore, if you are able to eat 1,800 calories a day to maintain your weight, your nutrient breakdown would look like this:

60 percent Complex Carbohydrates = 1,080 calories
15 percent Protein = 270 calories
25 percent Fat = 450 calories

An easy way to plan for this nutritional balance in your meals is to eat your evening meals each week according to the following schedule:

WEEKLY MAINTENANCE MEAL SCHEDULE
(Monday through Sunday)

Any two evening meals: Poultry
Any two evening meals: Pasta or Vegetable Dish
Any two evening meals: Fish
Any one evening meal: Lean Red Meat

GUIDELINE 2: Eat High-Fiber Foods Every Day

Foods that are high in dietary fiber (roughage) are essential to health and long-term weight maintenance. Fiber is that part of food that is not digestible. When fiber reaches your intestines it absorbs water and swells. This results in soft, bulky stools that move more quickly through your intestinal system.

Fiber in your diet can help prevent constipation and hemorrhoidal discomfort. In addition, many experts feel that dietary fiber reduces the risk of colon cancer.

Because fiber speeds the course of food through your body, your system will absorb fewer of the calories in those foods, helping you to control your weight.

A whole range of cereals, breads, vegetables, and fruits are high in fiber. Some of the best high-fiber choices include:

High-fiber cereal (for example, All-Bran)
Whole-wheat or rye bread
Bran muffins
Broccoli
Carrots
String beans
Brussels sprouts
Apples
Prunes
Oranges
Strawberries

It is still not clear exactly how much dietary fiber you should eat each day. Until scientists figure this out, eat plenty of high-fiber cereals, fruits, vegetables, and rye or whole-wheat bread. As you probably noticed, the Hilton Head Over-35 Diet is plentiful in these foods.

GUIDELINE 3: Eat Refined Sugar No More Than Two Times a Week

Sweets can have an obviously devastating effect on your efforts to maintain your weight. Not only are they high in calories but, even one cookie, candy bar, or piece of cake can entice you to have "just one more."

Of course, sugar is an ingredient in many things you eat. I am more concerned about the obvious sugar that you add to your coffee or that you eat in the form of desserts or snacks.

After completing the Hilton Head Over-35 Diet most people find that their desires for sweets are eliminated or greatly reduced. This is partly due to the nutritional composition of the diet and partly to the fact that the pattern of your sweet-eating habit has been broken.

If you do have cravings for sweets try to:

- Eat sweets (in moderation, of course) only out of the house at restaurants or at dinner parties. You will have more control over your sweets appetite if other people are around and will be less likely to "pig out."
- Never keep sweets in the house. If sweets are easily accessible you are more likely to be tempted by them. Studies have shown that the mere sight of sweets can trigger not only psychological cravings but physiological ones as well.
- Never eat sweets while alone or when you are emotionally upset. This is when you are more vulnerable to overindulging in sweets since you may use them for emotional solace and comfort. Develop healthier outlets for your emotional frustrations such as exercise, meditation, or "counseling" sessions with friends and loved ones.

GUIDELINE 4: Drink Plenty of Fluid

As you age your body is less sensitive to signals indicating increased fluid needs, so you must be sure to drink liquids every day. Don't rely on thirst to tell you whether to drink or not. Your goal should be to *drink four to six eight-ounce glasses of water or any noncaffeinated beverage each day*. Coffee, tea, and caffeinated soft drinks don't count since caffeine is a diuretic and robs your body of fluid.

GUIDELINE 5: Throw Out Your Salt Shaker

High sodium intake is associated with high blood pressure and excessive fluid retention. As you age these problems can become even more critical than when you were younger, so lowering the amount of salt you eat is important.

Your goal should be to reduce sodium consumption to 2,000 milligrams a day (about one teaspoon of table salt). Many people eat between 5,000 and 10,000 milligrams each day without realizing it. Many of the packaged and snack foods on the market contain such high levels of sodium that by eating even a little of them you get much more sodium than you need every day.

The easiest and best way for you to lower your sodium intake is to throw away your salt shaker. Whether you are home or eating out, never add salt to your food. After about a week you'll become accustomed to the new taste and you won't miss your salt one bit.

Many people at the Institute ask if I approve of salt substitutes. Most of these products contain potassium chloride. While a little extra potassium won't hurt you, you eat more than enough potassium naturally in fruits, vegetables, and potatoes. I would suggest you try a few herbs and spices as opposed to a salt substitute.

Don't Forget the Five Essential Rules

Although you will be eating more calories during maintenance than you did when you were losing weight, you must continue to stimulate your metabolism for the rest of your life. If you want to keep your metabolism strong, you must live by the Five Essential Rules of the Hilton Head Over-35 Diet that were given in chapter 7.

As a reminder, here are those rules as they apply to maintenance:

ESSENTIAL RULE 1: **You Must Eat Four Times a Day During the Week and Five Times a Day on Weekends**

ESSENTIAL RULE 2: **You Must Take Two Thermal Walks a Day**

ESSENTIAL RULE 3: **You Must Eat More Calories on Weekends Than You Do During the Week**

**NOTE: *During maintenance you should refer to your* total *calorie expenditure range (refer to chapter 6) to determine the number of weekday and weekend calories you should eat. You should eat the number of calories at the* low *end of this range on weekdays and the number of calories at the* high *end of your range on Saturday and Sunday. This means that you will be eating about 300 more calories each day on the weekend than you do during the week.*

ESSENTIAL RULE 4: **You Must Eat Mostly Grain-Based Foods, Starches, Vegetables, and Fruit**

ESSENTIAL RULE 5: **You Must Schedule the Muscle Reconditioners Three Times a Week to Strengthen Your Muscle Tissue**

By following these rules you will ensure that you will never regain your lost weight. Because your metabolism will be stronger than ever, you will have a much easier time controlling your weight. You will be able to eat a normal amount of food and even overindulge from time to time without paying the price on the scale.

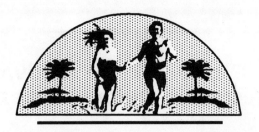

CHAPTER 15

The Hilton Head Motivational Plan

Having helped thousands of people to successfully lose weight, I realize that knowing how to diet is one thing while convincing yourself to begin dieting and to stick to it is quite another. Even though the Hilton Head Over-35 Diet is easy to follow, you may occasionally experience times when the stresses and strains of everyday life make it difficult to stay on the straight and narrow.

Well, don't worry a bit. You may have had motivational problems on other diets but not on this one. We have been studying motivation and habit change at the Hilton Head Health Institute for over a dozen years now. Based on these studies I have developed the Hilton Head Motivational Plan that will teach you how to become a *super-success*.

How I Discovered the Motivational Secrets of Dieting Success

A number of years ago, as part of our clinical follow-up program at the Hilton Head Health Institute, I began a series of in-depth interviews with what I call our *super-successes*. This group consisted of over-35 men and women who not only had successfully lost weight using the Hilton Head Over-35 Diet but had been able to keep their weight under control for many years. Now that's the true test of any diet system.

Most of these people had originally been about 30 pounds overweight but some had been very obese, weighing as much as 375 pounds. When I interviewed them they all were at their ideal weights and had been at that weight for an average of three years. They were all following the Five Essential Rules of the Hilton Head Over-35 Diet.

Interestingly enough, these successes seemed strangely unaware of the fact that they were following my plan so well. Not that they didn't consider it important or that they didn't feel pride in themselves. It's just that my rules had become so habitual, so much a part of their rejuvenated bodies and minds, they almost took their success for granted. In other words, they didn't give their new eating and exercise habits a second thought, they just knew what they had to do and they did it.

Let me tell you about Jane, a 37-year-old, overweight mother of two who never particularly liked to exercise. Not only did she successfully lose 28 pounds but she has kept those pounds off for two years. And in spite of her past dislike for exercise, Jane has not missed her morning thermal walk once in that entire two years. Now that's an accomplishment! When asked, "Why do you walk every morning at six-thirty?" she does not discuss diet or health reasons. Rather, her answer is extremely simple. "Because that's what I do at six-thirty every morning," is her reply. Her morning thermal walk has become so much a part of the new, younger Jane that having a conscious reason for walking is no longer necessary. It's a bit like brushing your teeth every day.

The Case of Dorothy

Dorothy is a 44-year-old travel agent from Maryland. She has been married to a building contractor for 23 years and has three teenage sons. Dorothy had a slight weight problem of five or ten excess pounds throughout her 20s but it was not until her mid 30s that she found her weight going up by leaps and bounds. When she enrolled at the Hilton Head Health Institute at age 39, Dorothy weighed 166 pounds. At five feet, five inches tall, she was at least 35 pounds overweight.

At that time Dorothy was depressed and disgusted with herself. She looked and felt old. She was even starting to act old. She always seemed to have aches and pains and was rarely happy. She had isolated herself by avoiding social and recreational activities. Nothing in her closet fit her and she couldn't stand the way she looked in her "fat" outfits.

To make matters worse Dorothy's husband watched everything she ate. He had little patience with her weight problem and continually blamed her for eating too much. Even her parents got into the act. Their favorite line was, "What a pretty face you have, Dorothy. If only you'd lose weight you'd be so attractive." These comments only served to anger and frustrate her.

It's not that Dorothy didn't try to diet. In fact, years ago she was good at dieting. She could lose weight on just about any diet. Unfortunately, the high-protein, low-carbohydrate diets and the fasting programs Dorothy used in the past had compounded her weight problem by slowing her metabolism. All of this made it more difficult for Dorothy to lose weight. She eventually gave up and lost all hope of ever losing weight.

When we tested her at the Institute we found that Dorothy

had too little muscle for her age. We convinced her that regular diets would simply not work for her over-35 metabolism. We gave her the hope that she needed. And, I am happy to report, Dorothy lost 38 pounds through the Hilton Head Over-35 Diet and, now, three years later, has continued to keep those 38 pounds off.

Recently, I interviewed her to see how she was doing. I can truly say that Dorothy looked and acted like a completely different person. She was vital and full of life.

Here's an excerpt from our conversation:

Dr. Miller: Dorothy, you are a genuine super-success at weight loss and habit change. Tell me what your experience has been like.

Dorothy: Well, as you know, Dr. Miller, I lost 38 pounds three years ago on the Hilton Head Over-35 Diet. My weight has not fluctuated more than three or four pounds since that time. I finally am free of my great burden. My weight had affected my whole life, even more than I realized. It was making me old before my time. I felt as though I had a fatal disease that was aging me more every day.

Dr. Miller: You sound like a different person than you did three years ago. What other changes have you experienced?

Dorothy: First of all, I like myself and feel good about myself. And, that wasn't just the result of losing weight. That was one of the new attitudes that helped me to be successful on your diet in the first place.

I feel younger, look younger, and am proud of my new image. I have more physical and mental energy than I've ever had before. I even enjoy taking my thermal walks every day. I look forward to my walking time because it's *my* time.

I'm also working again. As you know, I gave up working when my children were born and I had never gone back. Well, now, I have a career as a travel agent and I'm loving it. It gives me a real sense of purpose and accomplishment. Now I look forward to the challenges of my work *and* family life.

Dr. Miller: Speaking of your family, how do your husband and parents like the new you?

Dorothy: I'm not really sure and, in fact, it really doesn't matter to me. Oh, I'm sure they're pleased, but it doesn't concern me one way or the other. I don't mean to sound cold toward my family because I do love them.

You see, for the past several years, my family have been overly involved with my weight problem. And I always reacted by either going on some new, crazy fad diet to please them or by eating for spite to get back at them. Whenever they brought up the subject of my weight, I either felt frustrated, guilty, or just plain angry. It was like a game. So, as part of my new attitude, I decided not to play the game anymore.

If they were upset about my weight, that was their problem, not mine. And if they are pleased by my success, that's okay with me. Either way, it has no significance for me anymore. At your Institute, you convinced me that I had to be successful for me and nobody else.

Dr. Miller: So it was a completely different way of thinking, new attitudes that helped you put my Hilton Head Over-35 Diet into practice?

Dorothy: That's exactly right. You convinced me that the decision to look and feel years younger was mine. Well, I decided to make that decision and to take charge of my life. The realization that I had the ability to choose, the *power* to choose, made all the difference in the world.

You see, with the confidence I had in your Hilton Head Over-35 Diet I made a conscious decision to grab hold of the helm of my ship and do my own steering. The Hilton Head plan made so much sense. Instead of simply blaming me for my weight problem you explained what age had done to my metabolism and what I could do about it. Your approach is positive and it gave me something I could believe in. Now I believe in myself as well.

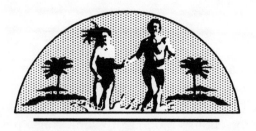

The Three Secrets of Motivational Success: How to "Rejuvenate" Your Mind As Well As Your Metabolism

If you want to reprogram your mind as well as your metabolism so that you achieve total revitalization, you must learn to live by my Three Secrets of Success. Remember, these are the secrets derived from people just like you. They once had an over-35 weight problem just like yours. However, they not only were able to lose their weight using the Hilton Head Over-35 Diet but, more important, they are keeping that weight off years later.

SECRET 1: ***PURPOSE:*** **You Must Develop a Purpose for Your Weight Loss That Has Personal Significance to You**

While your immediate goal is to speed up your metabolism so you can lose weight, you must also consider longer-term goals for your efforts. Sustained motivation in any endeavor comes not so much from achieving a particular goal but, rather, from *striving* for that goal. Because of this, your motivation to lose weight will be strongest in the beginning and the middle of your journey to attain your ideal weight. It will actually be the weakest when you finally reach your weight goal and just after that time.

I recently read about a man who set out on a journey to walk 1,900 miles from the southern tip of South America to the northernmost reaches of Canada. This arduous journey took six and a half years. At the very end, when he had reached his lifelong goal, his main emotion was depression rather than joy. He had accomplished his mission but lost his zeal.

This phenomenon is particularly common among creative people who often experience the same emotional trough after writing a novel, creating a masterful painting, or producing a play. Think back over your own life and I'm sure you'll find similar experiences.

Because of this, to attain maximum long-term commitment you must ask yourself the following question:

> *Once I start looking and feeling better, what will this enable me to do with my life?*

By viewing your goal in this way, once you attain your weight loss and younger body, you have not *completed* your self-change project, *you have only just begun.*

At the Hilton Head Health Institute I ask our participants to consider all of the possibilities that will be open to them once they are slim and feeling better. In fact, we ask each person to make a list of the ways in which their new bodies will change their lives. These changes don't have to be drastic. Often it's the most seemingly insignificant factors that have the most meaning. For example, one 55-year-old woman said that, once she lost her weight, her greatest dream was to dance with her husband without sweating profusely. Apparently the 25 pounds of excess fat she carried to the dance floor caused heavy perspiration that was extremely embarrassing to her.

You'll find that your slimmer body, younger appearance, increased stamina, and enhanced self-esteem will give you the physical ability and confidence to put your life in high gear. Now is the time to answer the question, "Once you look and feel better, what will this enable you to do with your life?" Consider a full range of activities, all the way from day-to-day practical ones such as buying a more attractive wardrobe to more challenging ones such as starting a new career.

Here are four steps to follow:

1. Sit back, close your eyes, and visualize yourself at your ideal weight, looking and feeling slim and vital.
2. Imagine what you would be doing from day to day, how you would be leading your life.
3. In a small notebook, write down all of the new activities that might be possible in your new life. Think of enjoyable activities that were part of your life when you were younger. Consider things you've always wanted to do but because of excuses (I'm too old, I'm too fat, I don't have the time, What would people say?) never attempted them.
4. Try out at least two or three activities on your list and see how you like them. Don't make excuses. Get started now.

This can be a fun exercise that will help to rejuvenate your mind as well as your body.

Try not to be too practical. Perhaps it's white-water rafting, or playing a role in a local theater production. Or perhaps you want to try a part-time job or even start your own business.

Once you've reached your weight goal don't let anything stop you from living life to the fullest.

SECRET 2: **BELIEF: You Must Believe That You Are Capable of Rejuvenating Your Metabolism, Losing Weight, and Changing Your Life**

Once you develop a purpose for your weight loss *you must believe that you are capable of achieving that success.* People who have lost weight and kept it off through the Hilton Head Over-35 Diet believe they have both the ability and the enduring commitment to manage their metabolism and weight permanently. They know they can master their age-related weight problem, not through magic, but through their own efforts. This expectation of success through personal effort is known as *self-mastery.* If you believe you will succeed and believe in the fact that your implementation of the Hilton Head Over-35 Diet will ensure your success, then you cannot fail. I have found that people who *believe* they will succeed put more effort into proving themselves right, especially when the going gets tough.

If you've had a history of failure at controlling your weight, you may be wondering how you can turn your negative experience into a new, positive conviction. I don't care how many times you've failed or how much self-doubt you have. Just because you failed at several attempts doesn't mean that you are a failure. It simply means your approach was wrong. Before now you didn't understand exactly how age affects your metabolism.

Of course, as we all know, success breeds success. The trouble is that when dieting, you may have a tendency to pay more attention to your failures than to your successes. I remember one particularly successful patient of mine named Janet who telephoned me one morning, sounding frantic. "Dr. Miller," she said, "I'm a failure. Last night I gave in and ate a whole pint of chocolate ice cream. I felt so frustrated and guilty this morning. Now I'll never be able to succeed."

Janet was labeling herself as a failure for one "slip," in spite of the fact that she had successfully resisted all sorts of temptations for the past six weeks. She had been and still is a true success story. However, at the time of the telephone call, Janet's interpretation of her "slip" led to a drop in her feelings of self-mastery. She almost had herself convinced that this one failure meant that she had lost her capacity to overcome future temptations.

I was able to help Janet by encouraging her to focus on all of the times in the past few weeks that she was tempted but had resisted the temptation. In fact, I had her describe these episodes in detail to me. I even had her write these positive self-mastery experiences in a notebook so she could give even more thought to them. In this way, Janet was finally convinced that her successes far outweighed her failures at sticking to nutrition and exercise rules.

The next time you have a problem with your feelings of confidence and self-mastery:

1. Review the past seven days in your mind.
2. Think of all the times you were tempted to eat high-calorie food but didn't and all of the times you didn't feel like taking your thermal walk but did anyway.
3. Write these episodes in a notebook, including as much detail as possible.
4. Pay particular attention to how you talked yourself into sticking to your commitment.

Another way to develop self-mastery is to become passionate about your commitment to changing the way you look and feel. Don't just brood over how fat you are, how old you are, or how many times you've failed at dieting. Confidence or lack of it is nothing more than what you are saying to yourself day after day. If you program your mind with insecurities and self-doubt, it will be programmed for failure. If you say to yourself, "I *will* succeed," rather than, "I hope this will work for me," your self-mastery will become stronger every day.

Your days of frustration, stagnation, and fat are over. You are too important for that. I want you to get angry. Not angry at yourself or anyone else. I want you to get mad at your weight problem, mad enough to take control of it and do something about it.

You don't have to put up with your weight or your sluggish metabolism anymore. You deserve a slimmer body and a more exciting life, and you're going to have both.

SECRET 3: *CONTROL:* You Must Believe That You and You Alone Are in Control of Your Life

This third Secret of Dieting Success is related to a psychological concept known as *locus of control*. This concept is concerned with the question, "Who do you believe is in control of your life?"

People who have an *external* locus of control believe that permanent weight loss is, for the most part, independent of their own efforts and is beyond personal control. They feel that the likelihood of lifelong weight changes is determined by a variety of external factors such as circumstances, chance, luck, doctors, and diet pills. In fact, once these "externals" hear that metabolism is a key factor in age-related weight gain, they may use metabolism as an excuse for being fat.

On the other hand, people who have an *internal* locus of control believe that their life as well as their metabolism and body weight is, to a large extent, under their personal control. Of course, they also realize that many factors such as circumstances, chance, and even age affect us all, *but only insofar as we allow them to affect us*.

Here's a good example. The "external" woman says, "My husband made me so angry last night. I went off my diet just to spite him. If he'd be less critical I would have an easier time losing weight." The "internal" woman views the same situation in these terms: "My husband made me so angry last night. I went off my diet just to spite him. *I* must find a way to deal more directly with his criticism and to keep myself from reacting to his comments by eating."

The "external" woman places the responsibility for her diet on her husband's shoulders. *He* must change his behavior before she can lose weight. She believes that she must wait for someone else to change before she can be successful. The "internal" woman, on the other hand, accepts responsibility for her own behavior regardless of what triggered it. She realizes that her husband's criticism is related to her eating but she sees it as her responsibility to do something about it. Either she must express her displeasure at his comments more directly, try to change his critical nature, or not allow her anger to sabotage her diet.

You can always tell an "external" by the way he or she refuses an offer of a dessert. The response is usually, "I'd love to have a piece but my doctor won't let me," or, "I'm not allowed to have that on my diet." The "internal" avoids excuses, takes full responsibility, and says, "No, thank you. I don't care for any." The correct idea here is not that you can't have dessert or that someone or something won't let you, but rather, *you are choosing not to have it.* Personal choice is a key element in the Hilton Head Over-35 Diet. Although there are nutritional and fitness rules you must live by, you must feel that you are choosing to abide by them rather than having them imposed on you. In this way, dieting is a series of important personal choices as opposed to negative control, confinement, and eventual diet rebellion.

Dieting doesn't have to be a control game. You simply have to make up your mind to change the control from external to internal. *You must become the master of your own destiny to ensure successful weight loss.*

If you are an "external" with an over-35 weight problem, you are probably waiting around for something to happen to enable you to lose weight. Maybe you're waiting for more time, less stress, more understanding, more insights into your psychological makeup. I say, stop waiting, because you're going to get fatter and older by the day. I say, now that I've given you the Hilton Head Over-35 Diet, it's time to get going. Take charge of your mind so you can take charge of your body!

Being All That You Can Be

I have found that without exception the super-successes I have interviewed are physically, intellectually, and creatively active. These successes are "on the go." They live by the motto that challenge, risk, and courage are absolutely necessary for a happy, fulfilling life.

One of my most successful cases is Bob, a 48-year-old marketing director who lost a total of 68 pounds on the Hilton Head Over-35 Diet. During one of his follow-up interviews three years after his weight loss, Bob talked about *his* "active" approach to life:

> Before you taught me the secrets of your motivational plan I used to sit passively, letting my life go by, allowing self-pity and depression to rule my life. I actually used my fat and my feelings about being middle-aged to keep my head buried in the sand. Now I look younger and feel great. I'm proud to be 48 years old and even prouder that I feel like 38. Now my life is full, not just with responsibilities, but with time for *me*.

The circular reasoning that comes from a passive attitude toward life can be a serious block to success at losing weight. One of my patients recalled how she used to say, "I can't lose weight because I'm too fat. It would be too difficult and take too long," and, "I can't play tennis at this weight. I'd be too embarrassed," and, "I can't go to parties and let people see me looking like this." She sat around passively, getting fatter and fatter and feeling older and older. She couldn't get active with her life because she was fat and she couldn't lose weight because she was inactive.

Super-successes have grown tired of waiting for the "right" time to lose weight, tired of waiting until the next Monday to start a diet or the next New Years' Day to make a commitment to exercise. They made a conscious decision to stop procrastinating and to stop using excuses. They began to take action, to get on the treadmill of life and run for all they're worth. They only wish they had started sooner.

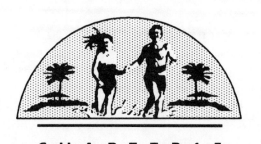

CHAPTER 17

A Final Word

You are now ready to start to feel younger than ever. The sooner you get started, the sooner you'll be able to enjoy your new slim, firm, youthful appearance. So, please don't procrastinate. Begin the Hilton Head Over-35 Diet immediately. It's so easy to put it off until next week or until you're not as busy. Now that you know what to do, now that you have hope that you can change your aging metabolism, get started!

Remember, I don't want you simply to lose weight. I want you to stimulate and revitalize your metabolism so you'll never have a weight problem again and you'll have a positive, youthful feeling about yourself for as long as you live.

The Hilton Head Over-35 Diet *will* work for you just as it has worked for the thousands of over-35 men and women who have attended the Hilton Head Health Institute. You *don't* have to be fat and frumpy as you age. You can stay thin and feel young as long as you follow my teachings. Every day I talk to people whose lives have been changed by this program. They lost fat, firmed up muscle, stimulated metabolic activity, and started to live their lives as if they were younger.

Don't let anyone discourage you or sidetrack you in your efforts. Don't believe anyone who tells you that you cannot speed up your metabolism. It's a proven fact that you can. Don't let anyone talk you into switching to some popular fad diet because it helped his Uncle Charlie lose 20 pounds. You need the Hilton Head Over-35 Diet to keep your metabolism young. Other diets will not have the same effect on your metabolism and may even slow it down. So ignore your friends and all their fad diets. Years from now you'll be slim and youthful and they'll be searching for another fad diet to rid them of their excess weight.

I have a great deal of faith in you. I know you will succeed. I want you to have a slimmer, healthier, and younger appearance as much as you do. As with all my patients, I am very interested in your success with the Hilton Head Over-35 Diet.

Please let me know how you are doing. I invite you to share your experiences on the diet with me. You can contact me by writing:

Hilton Head Health Institute
P.O. Box 7138
Hilton Head Island, SC 29938

Remember, don't hesitate. Start turning back your metabolic clock today!

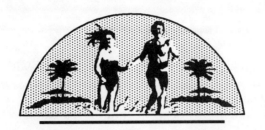

Hilton Head
Over-35 Diet
Recipes

Pasta

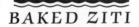

BAKED ZITI

Yield: 4 servings
280 calories per serving

8 ounces dry (4 cups cooked) ziti
1 teaspoon part-skim ricotta cheese
1 tablespoon chopped parsley
½ teaspoon nutmeg
2 cups Tomato Sauce, see page 203
4 tablespoons part-skim mozzarella cheese

1. Boil ziti until done.
2. Add to drained ziti the ricotta cheese, parsley, and nutmeg.

3. Place 1 cup ziti mixture in each bowl and top with ½ cup Tomato Sauce.
4. Sprinkle each with 1 tablespoon mozzarella cheese.
5. Place in oven at 400 degrees until mozzarella cheese is lightly browned.

CHEESE-FILLED MANICOTTA

**Yield: 225 calories
per manicotta**

1 manicotta
2½ tablespoons part-skim ricotta cheese
½ medium egg white
1 tablespoon Parmesan cheese
1 tablespoon parsley
Nutmeg (optional)
½ cup Tomato Sauce, see page 203

1. Parboil manicotta for 6 minutes.
2. Mix together ricotta cheese, egg white, Parmesan cheese, parsley, and nutmeg.
3. Fill manicotta with cheese mixture and cover with half of the Tomato Sauce.
4. Bake at 400 degrees for 30 minutes.

FETTUCCINE ALFREDO

Yield: 4 1-cup servings
260 calories per serving

½ pound fettuccine
1 teaspoon diet margarine
1 tablespoon skim milk
3 tablespoons low-fat vanilla yogurt
1 egg white
Freshly ground black pepper
2 tablespoons grated Parmesan cheese

1. Cook fettuccine *al dente*.
2. Place margarine in chafing dish.
3. Add fettuccine and toss gently until margarine is mixed with the noodles.
4. In a separate small bowl mix skim milk and yogurt so they are thoroughly blended. Add to fettuccine and toss.
5. Add egg white, pepper, grated cheese and toss once again.

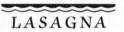

LASAGNA

Yield: 12 servings
250 calories per serving

1 pound dry lasagna
4 cups diced zucchini with skin on
1 cup thin-sliced mushrooms
4 cups Tomato Sauce, see page 203
3 cups low-fat cottage cheese
1 cup grated, low-fat mozzarella
4 tablespoons Parmesan cheese

1. Cook lasagna until noodles are chewy (about ¾ done).
2. Drain and cool.

3. Using a 10 × 12 × 3-inch baking dish or a layer-cake pan, place ⅓ of the noodles overlapping in the bottom of the pan.
4. Spread zucchini and mushrooms evenly over first layer of noodles.
5. Spread 2½ cups of the Tomato Sauce over zucchini and mushrooms.
6. Place another third of the noodles over the sauce.
7. Spread out evenly 3 cups low-fat cottage cheese.
8. Sprinkle the mozzarella cheese evenly over cottage cheese.
9. Place the rest of the noodles on the cheese.
10. Spread remaining 1½ cups sauce on the top.
11. Sprinkle with Parmesan cheese.
12. Cover with aluminum foil and bake in preheated 400-degree oven for ½ hour. Uncover and bake for ½ hour longer.

**NOTE: *Lasagna will be firmer and more tasteful if prepared, cooled, and reheated.*

LINGUINE WITH WHITE CLAM SAUCE

Yield: 4 servings
280 calories per serving

8 ounces uncooked linguine

Clam Sauce:
2 tablespoons vegetable oil
2 garlic cloves, chopped
2 shallots, chopped
½ cup fresh chopped parsley
½ cup white wine
1 cup chopped clams and juice
¼ cup freshly ground Parmesan cheese

1. Boil water for linguine.
2. Make the sauce: In the oil, sauté garlic, shallots, and parsley for 5 minutes. Add the wine and clams.
3. Cook the linguine *al dente*.

4. Pour sauce over linguini.
5. Add Parmesan cheese.
6. Toss and serve hot.

MACARONI AND CHEESE

Yield: 4 servings
200 calories per serving

1 ½ cups low-fat cottage cheese
½ cup skim or 1 percent milk
1 cup dry (2 cups cooked) elbow macaroni
2 tablespoons Parmesan cheese

1. In a blender, cream together the low-fat cottage cheese and milk.
2. Boil the elbow macaroni and rinse.
3. In a small ovenproof dish combine the macaroni with the cheese sauce.
4. Sprinkle top with Parmesan cheese.
5. Bake in preheated 400-degree oven for ½ hour.

MACARONI SUPREME

Yield: 4 servings
252 calories per serving

6 ounces or 1 ½ cups uncooked elbow macaroni
4 ounces ground chuck
1 cup Tomato Sauce, see page 203
4 teaspoons Parmesan cheese

1. Cook elbow macaroni in boiling water until tender and strain.
2. Cook ground beef; strain off fat.
3. In a saucepan, combine macaroni, beef, and Tomato Sauce, and heat until hot.
4. Top each serving with 1 teaspoon Parmesan cheese.

PASTA PRIMAVERA

Yield: 4 servings
200 calories per serving

6 ounces uncooked pasta swirls (rotini)
8 cherry tomatoes, halved
1 green pepper, julienned
½ cup onion, julienned
3 tablespoons Parmesan cheese
¼ cup sliced black olives
¼ cup low-calorie Italian dressing

1. Boil water and cook pasta *al dente*—rinse cold.
2. Prepare vegetables.
3. Put all ingredients in a mixing bowl and toss.
4. Serve immediately.

PASTA & VEGGIES I

Yield: 1 serving
350 calories

1½ ounces dry pasta (¾ cup cooked)
½ cup sliced mushrooms
½ cup sliced carrots
½ cup diced broccoli
½ cup plain yogurt
2 tablespoons Parmesan cheese
1 teaspoon corn-oil margarine

1. Cook pasta *al dente*.
2. Steam vegetables for 10 minutes.
3. Heat in a small saucepan the yogurt, Parmesan cheese, and margarine. Don't bring to a boil or the yogurt will separate.
4. Toss the vegetables and pasta together.
5. Place in a bowl and pour on sauce.
6. Serve hot.

PASTA & VEGGIES II

Yield: 1 serving
375 calories

2 ounces dry pasta (egg noodles)
½ cup sliced mushrooms
½ cup sliced yellow squash
½ cup sliced zucchini
½ cup sliced onions
2 teaspoons olive oil
1 clove fresh garlic, minced
1 tablespoon grated Parmesan cheese
Tomato wedge for garnish

1. Cook pasta *al dente*.
2. Sauté vegetables in 1 teaspoon olive oil with the garlic until tender (do not overcook).
3. Stir remaining oil into the pasta.
4. Pour vegetables over pasta.
5. Sprinkle on Parmesan cheese.
6. Garnish with tomato wedge—serve hot.

PIETRO'S PIZZA

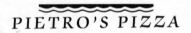

Yield: 1 pizza
500 calories

4 egg whites
1 whole egg
1 teaspoon baking powder
¼ cup all-purpose flour
¼ cup whole-wheat flour
¼ cup Tomato Sauce, see page 203
2 tablespoons grated, low-fat mozzarella cheese

1. Blend eggs, baking powder, and flours in a blender for 15 seconds.
2. Pour the mixture in 12-inch pan coated with vegetable spray coating.
3. Bake at 350 degrees for 12 minutes.
4. Remove and spread with Tomato Sauce and grated cheese.
5. Return to oven for 8 minutes.
6. Serve hot.

SPAGHETTI

Yield: 1 serving
195 calories per serving

¾ cup cooked spaghetti
½ cup Tomato Sauce, see page 203
1 tablespoon Parmesan cheese

1. Cook spaghetti in rapidly boiling water. Drain.
2. Place spaghetti in bowl and pour on Tomato Sauce.
3. Sprinkle with Parmesan cheese and serve.

TUNA-MUSHROOM CASSEROLE

Yield: 9 1-cup servings
192 calories per serving

4 cups cooked noodles or shells—2 cups dry weight
2 cups sliced mushrooms
½ cup diced onion
¼ cup reduced-calorie margarine
1 cup white wine
2 cups 1 percent or skim milk
½ cup flour dissolved in 1 cup water
8 ounces drained tuna fish packed in water
White pepper to taste

1. In a small frying pan sauté the mushrooms and onions in margarine until tender.
2. Place wine and milk in a saucepan and heat over medium heat.
3. When milk gets hot add the flour paste and beat with a whisk until blended.
4. Simmer for 5 minutes, stirring constantly, and remove from stove.
5. Mix in noodles, tuna, onions, mushrooms, and white pepper.
6. Pour into a small casserole dish and bake in a preheated 400-degree oven for 25–30 minutes.

VERMICELLI SCIACCA

Yield: 4 servings
250 calories per serving

½ pound vermicelli
2 tablespoons low-calorie corn-oil margarine
4 ounces part-skim ricotta cheese
2 tablespoons freshly chopped parsley
4 tablespoons freshly grated Parmesan cheese
Black pepper to taste

1. Cook vermicelli *al dente*.
2. Drain and place in warm bowl with 1 tablespoon of the margarine.
3. Melt remaining 1 tablespoon margarine in saucepan.
4. Stir in ricotta and stir until smooth.
5. Pour over vermicelli.
6. Sprinkle with parsley, Parmesan, and pepper.
7. Toss and serve—1 cup per person.

Fish

FISH CREOLE

Yield: 4 servings
215 calories per serving

4 5-ounce fish fillets
4 whole tomatoes, diced
2 cloves garlic, minced
1 green pepper, diced
½ cup diced green onion or ¼ cup diced shallots
1 teaspoon olive oil
1 bay leaf
1 lemon

1. Sauté prepared vegetables in olive oil until tender.
2. Broil or bake fish with lemon juice (squeeze ¼ lemon on each fillet).
3. Remove bay leaf, place fish on plates and top with vegetable mixture.
4. Serve immediately.

FLOUNDER WITH DILL SAUCE

Yield: 1 serving
145 calories per serving

2 tablespoons Dill Sauce, see page 199
4 ounces fresh flounder fillet

1. Heat prepared Dill Sauce slowly.
2. Broil fish for 5–8 minutes until firm.
3. Pour on 2 tablespoons Dill Sauce and serve.

FLOUNDER WITH LEMON MARGARINE

Yield: 2 servings
150 calories per serving

2 tablespoons low-calorie corn-oil margarine
1 fresh lemon
2 4-ounce flounder fillets

1. Melt margarine in saucepan.
2. Squeeze fresh lemon into margarine.
3. Spray a sheet pan with nonstick vegetable coating.
4. Place fillets on the pan.
5. Pour sauce over fish and bake at 400 degrees for about 5–8 minutes or until firm to the touch.
6. Serve immediately.

FROG LEGS PROVENÇALE

Yield: 1 serving
233 calories per serving

4 2-ounce frog legs
2½ tablespoons low-calorie margarine
1 tablespoon dry sherry or Chablis
1 tablespoon chopped parsley

1. Melt margarine in a nonstick medium frying pan.
2. Fry frog legs on medium heat until lightly brown on each side.
3. Add the sherry or Chablis and simmer for 2 minutes.
4. Sprinkle on parsley and serve.

SEAFOOD TETRAZZINI

Yield: 4 servings
360 calories per serving

½ pound uncooked spaghetti
½ cup chopped onion
2 teaspoons olive oil
2 cups low-sodium mushroom soup
1⅓ cups water
½ pound shrimp
2 tablespoons chopped parsley
2 teaspoons lemon juice
⅛ teaspoon each of thyme and marjoram
¼ cup grated Parmesan cheese

1. Cook spaghetti *al dente* and rinse.
2. In a large skillet sauté the onion in the olive oil.
3. Add the soup, water, shrimp, parsley, lemon juice, and spices.
4. Bring the sauce to a boil.
5. Put the sauce and spaghetti in a casserole dish.
6. Sprinkle with Parmesan cheese.
7. Heat under broiler and serve.

SHRIMP CURRY

Yield: 4 servings
265 calories per serving

20 ounces cooked shrimp
 3 tablespoons flour
 3 tablespoons low-calorie margarine
¼ cup Chablis
 1 pineapple ring, diced small
⅓ ripe banana, diced small
 1 tablespoon minced onion
 1 teaspoon curry powder
½ teaspoon mace
½ teaspoon thyme
 1 bay leaf
⅔ cup 1 percent or skim milk

1. Make a roux (flour-margarine mixture).
2. In a saucepan heat the wine, fruit, onion, and spices.
3. Simmer for 5 minutes.
4. Add the milk and bring to a simmer.
5. Add the roux and blend thoroughly.
6. Bring back to a simmer, stirring constantly.
7. Add shrimp and stir for 1 minute.
8. Serve on a bed of rice (calories not included).

SHRIMP NEWBURG

Yield: 1 serving
230 calories per serving

3 tablespoons Newburg Sauce, see page 201
5 ounces cooked and peeled medium shrimp

1. Prepare Newburg Sauce.
2. Prepare shrimp.
3. Pour hot Newburg Sauce over shrimp and serve immediately.

SHRIMP SCAMPI

Yield: 1 serving
295 calories per serving

5 ounces cooked and peeled large shrimp
5 tablespoons low-calorie margarine
1 clove garlic
½ slice low-calorie bread, grated

1. Slice cooked shrimp halfway up the back toward the tail.
2. Place shrimp upward so tails are touching in a flat, ovenproof dish.
3. Melt margarine in a small saucepan and squeeze the garlic into it.
4. Add the bread and mix.
5. Pour mixture over the shrimp and broil under broiler for about 2 minutes.
6. Serve immediately. (May be served on pasta or rice—calories not included.)

STUFFED FLOUNDER

Yield: 1 serving
297 calories per serving

5 ounces flounder fillet or any kind of whitefish
3 ounces fresh or frozen crabmeat
2 tablespoons low-calorie margarine

1. Cut flounder in half and place in a baking dish.
2. Place crabmeat on one piece of flounder.
3. Slice remaining piece of flounder in two lengthwise strips.
4. Place these pieces on each side of crabmeat.
5. Pour melted margarine over crabmeat and flounder.
6. Put a little water (1 or 2 tablespoons) in bottom of dish.
7. Broil until flounder turns white or bake at 475 degrees for 10 minutes.
8. Serve immediately.

STIR-FRY SHRIMP

Yield: 4 servings
200 calories per serving

1 tablespoon safflower oil
1 cup sliced carrots
1 cup diced scallions or sweet onion
1 cup diced broccoli
¼ cup water
1 tablespoon low-sodium soy sauce
12 ounces cooked peeled shrimp
1 cup sliced mushrooms
1 cup diced celery
1 cup halved cherry tomatoes
1 tablespoon cornstarch dissolved in ¼ cup cold water

1. Have all vegetables prepared and within hand's reach.
2. Heat wok to medium.
3. Add oil and carrots, and stir-fry for 3 minutes.
4. Add onions and broccoli, stir-fry for 3 more minutes.
5. Add ¼ cup water and soy sauce.
6. Bring to a boil and add the shrimp.
7. Add the mushrooms, celery, and cherry tomatoes.
8. Add the cornstarch and bring back to a boil, just until thickened.

Meat

BEEF BURGUNDY

Yield: 2 servings
285 calories per serving

8 ounces tender trimmed beef (fat off) cut in 1-inch cubes
1 small onion, minced
1 cup burgundy
1 bay leaf
1 cup fresh mushrooms sliced thin
2 tablespoons low-sodium tomato paste

1. Cook beef, onion, wine, and bay leaf in a frying pan for 10 minutes.
2. Add mushrooms and tomato paste.
3. Simmer 5 more minutes and serve.

BEEF KABOB

Yield: 1 serving
265 calories per serving

4 ounces cubed beef, preferably round steak or tenderloin, all fat removed
½ small onion cut in half again
¼ green bell pepper cut in 2 pieces
1 cherry tomato

1. Arrange beef cubes and cut-up vegetables on a skewer.
2. Broil until tender.
3. Serve with your favorite rice or pasta.

BEEF STROGANOFF

Yield: 4 servings
300 calories per serving

1 pound diced tenderloin or round steak
½ cup diced onions
1 clove garlic, minced
1 cup sliced mushrooms
1 tablespoon tomato paste
Pepper to taste
½ cup water
¼ cup cooking sherry
1 cup low-fat vanilla yogurt
1 cup cooked egg noodles

1. Sauté beef with onions and garlic.
2. When beef is browned add mushrooms, tomato paste, pepper, water, and sherry. Simmer for 5 minutes.
3. Remove from heat and stir in yogurt.
4. Pour over egg noodles and serve.

GRINGO'S GRUB

Yield: 4 servings
250 calories per serving

1 pound ground round or shredded beef
4 whole tomatoes, diced
2 medium onions, diced
4 fresh jalapeño peppers or 1 green bell pepper, diced
2 teaspoons garlic powder
2 tablespoons chili powder
½ teaspoon cayenne pepper (optional)

1. Cook ground beef and strain off fat.
2. In a frying pan add the vegetables, cooked ground beef, and spices.
3. Cook over high heat, stirring until hot.
4. Serve on a bed of rice (calories not included).

LAMB WITH MINT SAUCE

Yield: 4 servings
200 calories per serving

8 lean lamb chops
½ cup chopped fresh mint
4 individual packets (1-gram size) artificial sweetener
½ cup white vinegar

1. In a small saucepan combine mint, sweetener, and vinegar. Simmer for 5 minutes.
2. Place chops in a baking dish.
3. Pour sauce over chops.
4. Bake covered at 325 degrees for ½ hour or until chops are tender.
5. Serve immediately.

MOM'S MEAT LOAF

Yield: 4 servings
260 calories per serving

½ cup diced onion
½ cup diced green pepper
½ teaspoon hot sauce
2 teaspoons oregano
1 teaspoon garlic powder
2 teaspoons black pepper
½ cup water
1 pound ground round
4 egg whites

1. Cook onion, pepper, and spices in water in a frying pan until vegetables are tender.
2. Mix all ingredients together in a mixing bowl by hand.
3. Place in a small loaf pan or casserole dish.
4. Bake in preheated 400-degree oven for 20–30 minutes.
5. Slice in quarters and serve.

STEAK AU POIVRE

Yield: 2 servings
257 calories per serving

8 ounces trimmed rib eye, sirloin, or tenderloin, fat removed

2 tablespoons peppercorns

2 tablespoons Mustard Sauce, see page 201

1. Cut steak in two 4-ounce pieces.
2. Crush peppercorns with a rolling pin.
3. Coat the steaks with the fresh crushed peppercorns.
4. Broil to preferred doneness.
5. Pour Mustard Sauce on top and serve immediately.

TOURNEDOS ROSSINI

Yield: 2 servings
266 calories per serving

8 ounces beef tenderloin, fat removed

¼ cup Bordelaise Sauce, see page 197

1. Slice tenderloin against the grain into six small steaks.
2. Prepare Bordelaise Sauce.
3. Sauté the steaks using vegetable spray coating in a nonstick frying pan.
4. Pour hot sauce over steaks and serve.

VEAL PICCATA

Yield: 4 servings
275 calories per serving

This recipe can also be prepared using 1 pound of skinless chicken breast fillets instead of the veal.

1 pound boneless veal steaks, fat removed
½ cup whole-wheat flour
2 tablespoons parsley
2 tablespoons plus 1 teaspoon low-calorie margarine
Juice of 1 lemon

1. Cut veal steak in four 4-ounce pieces.
2. Pound out each piece of veal with a hand meat tenderizer (hammer).
3. Mix the flour and parsley together and pour on a flat plate.
4. Melt margarine in a nonstick frying pan and add the lemon juice.
5. Dust each side of the veal steaks with the flour-parsley mixture.
6. Fry the veal steaks on each side in the melted margarine.

VEAL ROLLETTES

Yield: 4 servings
150 calories per serving

8 ounces boneless veal steaks, fat removed
4 large asparagus spears
2 slices of your favorite low-calorie cheese

1. Cut and trim veal into four 2-ounce pieces.
2. Pound out each piece of veal with hand meat tenderizer (hammer).
3. Roll up in veal an asparagus spear and half a slice of cheese.
4. Secure with a toothpick.

5. Spray small oven pan with vegetable spray coating.
6. Place veal in pan with toothpick facing up.
7. Bake in preheated 400-degree oven for 12–18 minutes.

Poultry

CHICKEN À LA KING

Yield: 4 servings
285 calories per serving

 1 pound diced skinned, boneless chicken breast
2½ cups water
 3 tablespoons low-calorie margarine
 3 tablespoons flour
 ½ cup sliced mushrooms
 ½ cup diced pimento
 ½ cup diced green pepper
 ½ cup diced onions

1. Boil chicken in the water for 10 minutes.
2. While chicken is boiling, cook the roux (margarine and flour) for 5 minutes.
3. Add the vegetables to the cooked chicken.
4. Stir in the roux and cook for 10 minutes, stirring occasionally.
5. Serve over noodles or rice (calories not included).

CHICKEN CACCIATORE

Yield: 2 servings
275 calories per serving

2 4-ounce raw chicken breast fillets or skinned breast with bone
½ cup sliced mushrooms
1 small onion, minced
1 medium bell pepper, diced
½ cup burgundy
1 cup Tomato Sauce, see page 203

1. Combine all ingredients in a skillet or frying pan, cover, and simmer for 20–30 minutes.
2. Place chicken on a plate and pour the hot sauce and vegetables over the breasts.
3. Serve with your favorite pasta (calories not included).

CHICKEN (TURKEY) HASH

Yield: 4 servings
250 calories per 4-ounce serving

1½ cups Chicken (turkey) Stock (see page 198)
16 ounces cooked chicken (turkey), diced
2 small whole onions, chopped
3 celery stalks, chopped
2 medium green peppers, chopped
½ teaspoon thyme

1. Add diced chicken (turkey) and all other ingredients to prepared stock in pot.
2. Cook on high heat for 5 minutes; reduce to low heat, and cook 40 minutes.

CHICKEN PARMESAN

Yield: 2 servings
275 calories per serving

2 4-ounce raw skinned and boned chicken breasts
½ cup Tomato Sauce, see page 203
2 ounces low-fat mozzarella cheese

1. Place chicken breasts in a small skillet sprayed with vegetable spray.
2. Pour Tomato Sauce over chicken.
3. Place 1 ounce of cheese on each piece.
4. Simmer covered for 10 minutes.
5. Serve immediately.

COQ AU VIN

Yield: 2 servings
265 calories per serving

½ clove garlic
1½ cups red burgundy
1 small onion, julienned
1 bay leaf
½ teaspoon thyme
2 large chicken breasts, skinned, with bone
1 cup mushroom caps
2 tablespoons cornstarch
¼ cup cold water

1. Place garlic, burgundy, onion, bay leaf, and thyme in a small skillet or frying pan.
2. Bring to a boil and let simmer 5 minutes.
3. Add chicken and mushrooms and continue to simmer, 45 minutes.
4. Remove garlic clove.
5. Dissolve cornstarch in water and stir into sauce.

6. Place chicken on a plate.
7. Pour sauce and vegetables over chicken, and serve.

ITALIAN CHICKEN I

Yield: 2 servings
290 calories per serving

2 4-ounce raw skinned and boned chicken breasts
2 tablespoons low-calorie margarine
1 teaspoon granulated garlic
1 teaspoon oregano
1 teaspoon basil
1 tablespoon water
1-ounce slice, low-fat mozzarella cheese

1. Melt margarine with spices and water in a small frying pan or skillet.
2. Add chicken, cover, and simmer for 15 minutes.
3. Add cheese and continue to simmer uncovered until cheese has melted.
4. Serve immediately.

ITALIAN CHICKEN II

Yield: 2 servings
250 calories per serving

2 4-ounce raw skinned and boned chicken breasts
¼ cup low-calorie Italian dressing
1 teaspoon granulated garlic
1 teaspoon oregano
1 teaspoon basil
1 tablespoon Parmesan cheese

1. Place dressing and spices in a small frying pan or skillet.
2. Add chicken.

3. Sprinkle Parmesan cheese on top of chicken.
4. Simmer covered for 15–20 minutes, and serve.

JAMAICAN CHICKEN

Yield: 2 servings
250 calories per serving

2 4-ounce raw chicken breasts, skinned
2 pineapple slices
1 teaspoon instant coffee dissolved in 1 tablespoon hot water
½ cup low-fat vanilla yogurt

1. Place chicken in a small baking dish.
2. Stir dissolved coffee into the yogurt.
3. Pour yogurt over chicken and place pineapple on top.
4. Bake in preheated 350-degree oven for 30–40 minutes. May also be sautéed in a small skillet.

LADY DAPHNE'S CHICKEN

Yield: 1 serving
250 calories per serving

1 medium chicken breast (about 3 ounces of meat)
½ teaspoon rosemary
1 tablespoon vanilla yogurt

1. Remove skin from chicken and place in ungreased baking pan.
2. Bake 30 minutes at 350 degrees.
3. Remove from oven and cover with yogurt.
4. Sprinkle top with rosemary leaves.
5. Return to oven for 15 minutes before serving.

MEXICAN CHICKEN

Yield: 2 servings
260 calories per serving

2 4-ounce skinned, boned chicken breast halves
1 small jalapeño pepper, diced
1 tablespoon chili powder
1 cup Tomato Sauce, see page 203

1. Add jalapeño pepper and chili powder to Tomato Sauce.
2. Place chicken with sauce in a small skillet or frying pan; cover.
3. Simmer for 20–30 minutes.
4. Serve chicken with sauce on top.

QUICKY CHICKY BLUE

Yield: 2 servings
250 calories per serving

2 4-ounce skinned raw chicken breasts
¼ cup commercially prepared, diet blue cheese dressing
2 teaspoons chopped parsley

1. Place chicken in a small skillet or frying pan.
2. Add a little water to bottom of pan.
3. Pour blue cheese dressing over chicken.
4. Sprinkle with parsley.
5. Simmer, covered, for 15–20 minutes.

STIR-FRY CHICKEN

Yield: 4 servings
275 calories per serving

1 tablespoon safflower oil
1 pound raw chicken breasts or boneless chicken, skinned and diced
1 cup sliced mushrooms
1 cup diced broccoli
¼ cup diced onion
1 carrot, sliced
1 cup pea pods
1 cup sliced yellow squash
¼ cup water
1 tablespoon cornstarch dissolved in additional ¼ cup cold water
1 tablespoon low-sodium soy sauce

1. Have all ingredients ready to cook.
2. Heat wok to medium heat, about 300 degrees.
3. Add oil and chicken and stir-fry for 30 seconds.
4. Raise heat to high, add all the vegetables and water, and stir-fry for 2 minutes.
5. Add the dissolved cornstarch and soy sauce.
6. Stir-fry for 1 minute.
7. Serve immediately.

Vegetables

CURRIED RICE

Yield: 3 servings
50 calories per ½ cup serving

½ cup uncooked brown or wild rice
½ cup chicken stock
½ cup water
1 teaspoon curry powder

1. Place ingredients in a saucepan.
2. Bring to a boil and let simmer 30 minutes or until rice is fluffy.
3. May also be done in the oven at 400 degrees.

Options: If you don't like curry you may use parsley or your favorite spice.

HOT VEGETABLE PLATE

Yield: 1 serving
230 calories

½ cup asparagus
½ cup broccoli
½ cup yellow squash
½ cup zucchini
½ cup sliced carrots
2 tablespoons low-calorie margarine
2 teaspoons lemon juice
1 tablespoon Parmesan cheese

1. Steam the vegetables to desired doneness.
2. Melt the margarine in a saucepan and add lemon juice.
3. Add the steamed vegetables and toss.
4. Place vegetables on a plate.
5. Sprinkle with Parmesan and serve immediately.

MELANIE'S POTATOES

Yield: 4 servings
120 calories per serving

4 medium potatoes
¼ cup minced shallots
½ cup diced mushrooms
1 tablespoon fresh chopped parsley
¼ cup skim milk

1. Peel potatoes and prepare vegetables.
2. Boil potatoes for about 30 minutes.
3. Mix all ingredients together.
4. Heat and serve.

ROASTED CHIPS

Yield: 2 servings
45 calories per serving

1. Cut whole baking potato lengthwise in eighths like large french fries.
2. Bake in oven on a cookie sheet for ½ hour at 400 degrees.
3. Serve hot.

SQUASH CASSEROLE

Yield: 2 servings
40 calories per serving

1 cup sliced yellow squash
1 tablespoon chopped onion
2 tablespoons low-fat cottage cheese
¼ teaspoon caraway seeds
1 teaspoon grated Parmesan cheese
Freshly ground black pepper

1. Steam or boil squash and onion until tender. Do not overcook.
2. Drain and mix in cottage cheese, caraway seeds, and pepper.
3. Place in baking dish and sprinkle top with Parmesan cheese. Bake at 350 degrees for 30 minutes.

STEWED TOMATOES

Yield: 2 servings
25 calories per serving

1 cup chopped tomatoes
1 tablespoon chopped onions
1 tablespoon chopped green pepper
¼ teaspoon oregano
¼ teaspoon basil
¼ teaspoon artificial sweetener

1. Cook vegetables and spices in saucepan with 2 tablespoons water until tender.

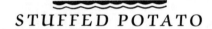

STUFFED POTATO

Yield: 2 servings
90 calories per serving

1 medium potato (5 ounces)
½ cup low-fat cottage cheese
1 teaspoon chives

1. Bake the potato at 400 degrees for 40 minutes.
2. Cut potato in half while hot and scoop out insides of potato into bowl.
3. Blend cottage cheese in blender or mixer until smooth.
4. Mix potato insides and cottage cheese.
5. Refill potato skin.
6. Bake at 350 degrees for 20 minutes.
7. Serve hot.

VEGETABLE MÉLANGE

Yield: 4 servings
145 calories per serving

2 cups broccoli
2 cups cauliflower
2 cups carrots, sliced thin
½ cup sweet onion, julienned
2 cups green beans
½ cup low-calorie Italian dressing
3 tablespoons Parmesan cheese

1. Steam the vegetables for about 10 minutes.
2. Divide vegetables into four bowls.
3. Pour 2 tablespoons Italian dressing over each and sprinkle with Parmesan cheese.
4. Serve immediately.

JAMBALAYA

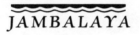

Yield: 4 servings
170 calories per serving

2 cups sliced mushrooms
2 medium diced green peppers
1 rib diced celery
2 diced pimentos
4 chopped tomatoes
¼ cup corn-oil margarine
1 cup cooked rice
   Pinch of cayenne pepper
¼ teaspoon paprika

1. Sauté the vegetables in one tablespoon of the corn-oil margarine.

2. Add remaining ingredients to vegetables and sauté for about 10 minutes more.
3. Serve immediately.

Salads

CHICKEN SALAD

Yield: 1 serving
250 calories per serving

2 ounces diced cooked chicken meat
½ diced apple
½ cup diced celery
¼ diced onion
1 tablespoon low-calorie mayonnaise
1 whole medium tomato

1. Place chicken, apple, celery, and onion in a mixing bowl and toss gently.
2. Add mayonnaise and toss gently.
3. Slice the tomato nearly all the way through in sixths.
4. Open up and stuff with the chicken salad.
5. Serve on a bed of lettuce.

COLD STUFFED TOMATO

Yield: 1 serving
160 calories per serving

1 whole medium tomato
½ cup regular cottage cheese
1 teaspoon chives
White pepper to taste

1. In a small bowl mix cottage cheese, chives, and pepper to taste.

2. Core the tomato and slice nearly all the way through from the top into sixths.
3. Open up and stuff with the cottage-cheese mixture.
4. Serve on a bed of lettuce.

CRABMEAT SALAD

Yield: 1 serving
245 calories per serving

4 ounces cooked, drained crabmeat
½ cup diced celery
   Juice of ½ lemon
1 tablespoon low-calorie mayonnaise
   White pepper to taste
1 tomato

1. Toss the crabmeat and celery gently together in a mixing bowl with the lemon juice.
2. Add the mayonnaise and white pepper and mix gently.
3. Place on a lettuce leaf with the tomato cut into wedges, or stuff the whole tomato.
4. To stuff, slice the tomato nearly all the way through in sixths.

HAWAIIAN COLE SLAW

Yield: 4 servings
35 calories per ½ cup serving

2 cups finely shredded cabbage
½ cup crushed pineapple (packed in water)
2 tablespoons low-calorie mayonnaise
2 tablespoons red wine vinegar
1 teaspoon celery seed

1. Mix all ingredients together and chill.
2. Serve with your favorite seafood.

MACARONI SALAD

Yield: 4 servings
135 calories per serving

4 ounces dry macaroni
1 stalk diced celery
1 tablespoon grated carrot
¼ cup diced onion
1 tablespoon diced pimentos
8 halved cherry tomatoes
2 teaspoons low-calorie salad dressing

1. Cook pasta in boiling water until *al dente*.
2. Rinse macaroni.
3. Mix all ingredients in a mixing bowl.
4. Chill and serve.

PETER'S POTATO SALAD

Yield: 4 servings
75 calories per 1 cup serving

3 cups cooked potatoes, diced
4 cooked egg whites, diced small
1 stalk celery, diced
¼ cup diced onion
¼ cup low-calorie mayonnaise
1 teaspoon dry mustard
1 teaspoon celery seed
  White pepper to taste
1 tablespoon red wine vinegar
  Paprika

1. Combine all ingredients except paprika and toss gently until mixed well.

2. Chill and place on a bed of lettuce.
3. Serve with paprika sprinkled on top.

PLAIN JAIN'S COLE SLAW

Yield: 4 servings
15 calories per ½ cup serving

2 cups finely chopped cabbage
1 carrot, shredded
¼ cup red wine vinegar
½ teaspoon garlic powder
½ teaspoon dill weed
1 teaspoon celery seed
½ teaspoon ground pepper
   Artificial sweetener to taste

1. Mix all ingredients together thoroughly by hand.
2. Chill and serve.

SHRIMP AND CUCUMBER SALAD

Yield: 4 cups
145 calories per cup

10 ounces peeled salad shrimp
1 cup diced cucumber
¼ cup diced onion
½ cup diced celery
1 tablespoon diced pimento
1 tablespoon chopped parsley
½ cup chopped green pepper
¼ cup low-calorie mayonnaise
   White pepper to taste

1. Cook shrimp in boiling water and cool.
2. Mix together the shrimp and all other ingredients.
3. Chill and serve on a bed of lettuce.

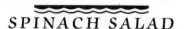

SHRIMP AND MACARONI SALAD

Yield: 4 servings
175 calories per 1 cup serving

1 cup uncooked (2 cups cooked) elbow macaroni
1 cup cooked salad shrimp
¼ cup low-calorie mayonnaise
¼ cup diced onion
½ cup diced celery
1 teaspoon dry mustard
White pepper to taste

1. Boil the macaroni, rinse under cold water, and drain well.
2. Mix together all ingredients and chill.
3. Serve on a bed of lettuce.

SPINACH SALAD

Yield: 1 serving
170 calories per serving

1 cup fresh spinach
¼ cup sliced fresh mushrooms
5 raw onion rings
1 whole hard boiled egg, sliced
1 whole tomato, cut in quarter wedges
2 tablespoons low-calorie dressing

1. Rinse and tear up spinach.
2. Place spinach on a plate and cover with mushrooms, onions, sliced egg, and tomato wedges.

3. Pour dressing on top.
4. Serve with melba toast.

TUNA SALAD

Yield: 4 servings
140 calories per 4-ounce serving

1 pound water-packed tuna, drained
¼ cup diced celery
¼ cup diced onion
2 tablespoons low-calorie mayonnaise
½ teaspoon thyme

1. Mix all ingredients.
2. Serve with tomato and cucumber slices.

Sauces

À LA KING SAUCE

Yield: 3 cups
120 calories per ½ cup

An excellent choice for poultry.

½ cup diced green peppers
½ cup fresh sliced mushrooms
¼ cup diced onion
¼ cup diced pimentos
2 tablespoons low-calorie margarine
2 tablespoons dry sherry
2 cups White Sauce, see page 203

1. Sauté vegetables in the margarine.
2. Add sherry and simmer 5 minutes.
3. Add White Sauce and simmer 2 more minutes.

BARBECUE SAUCE

Yield: 1 cup
20 calories per tablespoon

A favorite for outdoor cooking.

1 cup Tomato Sauce, see page 203
Juice of ½ lemon
1 tablespoon Worcestershire sauce
2 tablespoons white vinegar
1 garlic clove, minced or pressed
1 bay leaf
1 teaspoon chili powder
3 tablespoons honey
½ teaspoon liquid smoke (optional)

1. Combine all ingredients in a saucepan and simmer for ½ hour or until sauce thickens.
2. Cook on your favorite meat or poultry.

BEEF STOCK

Yield: 2 quarts
Calories: 25 calories per cup

The finished stock may be frozen.

2 pounds beef bones
1 medium onion, quartered
2 quarts water
3 carrots, quartered
3 celery stalks, quartered

1. Pour 1 cup water in bottom of a roasting pan and add the bones and vegetables.
2. Bake in preheated 450-degree oven, tossing occasionally until bones brown.
3. Remove from oven and pour all ingredients into a stockpot or saucepan.
4. Put 2 quarts of water into the roasting pan and bring to a boil on top of stove, scraping everything off the sides and bottom.
5. Pour everything into the stockpot and simmer uncovered for 2 hours.
6. Strain through colander or cheesecloth.
7. Chill and remove, then discard any fat that forms on the top.

BORDELAISE SAUCE

Yield: 2 cups
13 calories per tablespoon

Good for steaks and meat loaves.

½ cup sliced mushrooms
2 tablespoons low-calorie margarine
½ cup dry red wine
1 teaspoon parsley
1 garlic clove, minced or pressed
1 cup Brown Sauce, see recipe below

1. Sauté sliced mushrooms in the margarine.
2. Add mushrooms, red wine, parsley, and garlic to the Brown Sauce.
3. Simmer 2 minutes to blend.

BROWN SAUCE

Same procedure as White Sauce, see page 203, using browned flour or a brown stock. Browned flour is white flour browned in a frying pan. Do not burn.

CHICKEN STOCK

Yield: 2 quarts
Calories: 25 calories per cup

The finished stock may be frozen.

3 pounds leftover chicken parts (neck, wings, bones, etc.)
2 medium onions, quartered
4 celery stalks, diced large
4 carrots, diced large
1 bay leaf
2 quarts water
2 egg shells

1. Place all ingredients in a stockpot and simmer for 2 hours.
2. Strain through colander or cheesecloth.
3. Refrigerate.
4. When stock cools, fat will rise to the top and should be removed and discarded.

CLOSE COCKTAIL SAUCE

Yield: 1 cup
10 calories per tablespoon

3 tomatoes
2 tablespoons horseradish
1 tablespoon tomato paste
1 teaspoon lemon juice

1. Peel tomatoes.
2. Put all ingredients in a blender and purée.
3. Place in saucepan and simmer for 15 minutes.
4. Chill before serving.

DILL SAUCE

Yield: 18 tablespoons
15 calories per tablespoon

A tangy sauce for fish.

1 cup low-fat plain yogurt
2 tablespoons prepared horseradish
1 teaspoon dry mustard
1 tablespoon dillweed

1. Blend all ingredients together by hand.
2. Heat on low heat and serve.

FLORENTINE SAUCE

Yield: 18 tablespoons
15 calories per tablespoon

A complementary fish sauce.

¼ cup dry white wine
　Dash hot sauce
¼ teaspoon oregano
½ teaspoon dillweed
½ teaspoon white pepper
1 cup White Sauce, see page 203

1. Add wine and seasonings to White Sauce and simmer for 2
minutes.
2. Serve on your favorite fish with ½ cup steamed spinach.

MINT SAUCE

Yield: 1 cup
25 calories per tablespoon

This goes well with lamb.

1 cup white vinegar
1 tablespoon fresh mint leaves
1 tablespoon cornstarch
Low-calorie sweetener of your choice

1. Mix all ingredients together in a small saucepan and simmer 15 minutes.

MOCK SOUR CREAM

Yield: 1¼ cups
11 calories per tablespoon

1 cup low-fat cottage cheese
¼ cup skim or 1 percent milk
2 teaspoons lemon juice

1. Place all ingredients in a mixer and blend until smooth and creamy.

MUSTARD SAUCE

Yield: 18 tablespoons
17 calories per tablespoon

Tasty with beef or fish.

1 cup White Sauce, see page 203
1 tablespoon low-sodium mustard
1 tablespoon white vinegar
   White pepper to taste

1. In a small saucepan, combine White Sauce with remaining ingredients.
2. Simmer for 2 minutes and serve.

NEWBURG SAUCE

Yield: 18 tablespoons
18 calories per tablespoon

A flavorful seafood sauce.

1 cup White Sauce, see page 203
2 tablespoons sherry
1 teaspoon low-calorie margarine
1 teaspoon paprika
   White pepper to taste

1. In a small saucepan, combine White Sauce with sherry, margarine, and spices.
2. Simmer for 2 minutes and serve.

ORANGE SAUCE

Yield: ¾ cup
25 calories per tablespoon

Great for fowl and poultry.

Juice from 4 oranges
1 tablespoon grated orange peel
2 tablespoons honey
1 tablespoon cornstarch
2 tablespoons cold water

1. Heat orange juice, orange peel, and honey in a small saucepan.
2. Dissolve cornstarch in water.
3. Add cornstarch to saucepan and simmer for 5 minutes.
4. Serve on your favorite fowl.

RAISIN SAUCE

Yield: 1 cup
15 calories per tablespoon

An excellent poultry sauce.

2 tablespoons raisins
1 cup unsweetened apple juice
1 tablespoon honey
1 tablespoon cornstarch dissolved in 1 tablespoon cold water

1. In a small saucepan, mix together raisins, apple juice, and honey.
2. Bring to a boil and let simmer 5 minutes.
3. Stir in cornstarch mixture and simmer for another minute.
4. Serve on your favorite poultry.

TOMATO SAUCE

Yield: 5 cups
100 calories per cup

10 medium tomatoes
 1 cup diced onion
 8 cloves garlic, minced
¼ cup Beef Stock (see page 196)
 3 tablespoons oregano
 1 tablespoon basil
 1 bay leaf
 1 teaspoon thyme
   Black pepper to taste
½ cup low-sodium tomato paste
¼ cup burgundy
   Artificial sweetener to taste

1. Place tomatoes in a pot, cover with water, and heat until skins loosen.
2. Peel tomatoes and purée in a blender. Place tomatoes in a heavy sauce pot or frying pan.
3. Sauté together onion, garlic, and Beef Stock in a nonstick frying pan.
4. Add onion mixture and spices to the tomatoes and simmer on medium heat for ½ hour.
5. Add tomato paste, wine, artificial sweetener, and simmer for ½ hour more.

WHITE SAUCE

Yield: 18 tablespoons
25 calories per tablespoon

2 tablespoons low-calorie margarine
2 tablespoons all-purpose flour
1 cup 1 percent or skim milk or clear stock

1. Melt margarine in small saucepan.
2. Add flour and cook for about 3 minutes, stirring constantly.
3. Heat milk or stock in another saucepan.
4. Combine flour mixture and heated milk or stock, and blend well.
5. Bring to a boil and remove from stove.

Miscellaneous

BAKED APPLE

Yield: 1 serving
80 calories

1 fresh apple
1 teaspoon cinnamon
1 teaspoon nutmeg

1. Core apple.
2. Put cinnamon and nutmeg in the core.
3. Bake uncovered at 350 degrees for 30 minutes.

Options: You may add yogurt or raisins after baking to make a fine dessert.

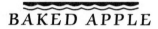

EGG-WHITE OMELET

Yield: 1 serving
145 calories

3 egg whites
¼ cup cottage cheese*
¼ cup Tomato Sauce (see page 203)
1 teaspoon Parmesan cheese

1. Heat a small egg pan or electric omelet pan.
2. Beat egg whites.
3. Spray hot pan with vegetable coating.
4. Pour in eggs; spread egg whites evenly in pan.
5. Spread cottage cheese over half the eggs.
6. Fold over other half of eggs.
7. Place on an ovenproof plate.
8. Top with Tomato Sauce and Parmesan cheese.
9. Place under broiler for 1 minute.
10. Serve immediately.

*You may use ½ cup combination of spinach, mushrooms, and onion in place of the cottage cheese. Sauté the vegetables in 1 teaspoon corn-oil margarine before adding to omelet.

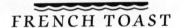

FRENCH TOAST

Yield: 4 slices
60 calories per slice

8 egg whites
¼ cup skim or 1 percent milk
2 teaspoons cinnamon
1 teaspoon vanilla extract
4 slices low-calorie regular or wheat bread

1. Place egg whites in a bowl.
2. Add milk, cinnamon, and vanilla.
3. Beat with a whip or blender.
4. Heat Teflon pan or griddle.
5. Spray with vegetable spray coating.
6. Coat bread with egg mixture and fry on each side until browned.
7. Serve with your favorite low-calorie syrup.

FRUIT AMBROSIA

Yield: 1 serving
100 calories

Juice of 1 lemon
½ apple, finely chopped
½ orange, finely chopped
½ grapefruit, finely chopped
8 seedless grapes
¼ honeydew, finely chopped
¼ cantaloupe, finely chopped
Grated coconut

1. Combine ingredients except coconut in mixing bowl and chill.
2. Sprinkle lightly with grated coconut.

LOW-CAL CRANBERRY JELLY

Yield: 8¼-cup servings
10 calories per ¼ cup

1½ cups fresh cranberries
2½ cups water
1 envelope Orange D-Zerta with Nutra-Sweet
5 packets artificial sweetener

1. Boil the cranberries in the water for 20 minutes.
2. Remove from stove and mash the cranberries while they are still in the water.
3. Add the gelatin and sweetener.
4. Chill in desired container.
5. Serve when set.

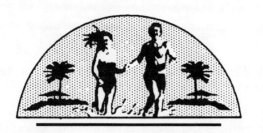

APPENDIX B
Scientific
Bibliography

Briggs, G. M., and Calloway, D. H. *Nutrition and Physical Fitness*. Philadelphia: W. B. Saunders Company, 1979.

Cioffi, L. A.; James, W. P. T.; and Van Itallie, T. B. (eds.). *The Body Weight Regulatory System: Normal and Disturbed Mechanisms*. New York: Raven Press, 1981.

Davis, J. M.; Sadri, S.; Sargent, R. G.; and Ward, D. "Thermogenic Effects of Pre-Prandial and Post-Prandial Exercise." *Addictive Behaviors*, in press.

Garrow, J. S. *Energy Balance and Obesity in Man*. Amsterdam: Elsevier/North Holland Biomedical Press, 1978.

Keys, A.; Taylor, H. L.; and Grande, F. "Basal Metabolism and Age of Adult Man." *Metabolism* 22, 579–87, 1973.

McArdle, W. D.; Katch, F. I.; and Katch, V. L. *Exercise Physiology: Energy, Nutrition, and Human Performance*. Philadelphia: Lea & Febiger, 1981.

Miller, P. M. *The Hilton Head Metabolism Diet.* New York: Warner Books, 1983.

Miller, W. J., and Stephens, T. "The Prevalence of Overweight and Obesity in Britain, Canada, and the United States." *American Journal of Public Health* 77, 1, 38–41, 1987.

Segal, K. R., and Gutin, B. "Thermic Effects of Food and Exercise in Lean and Obese Women." *Metabolism* 32, 581–89, 1983.

Stock, M., and Rothwell, N. *Obesity and Leanness: Basic Aspects.* London: John Libbey & Co., 1982.

Wadden, T. A., and Stunkard, A. J. "Psychopathology and Obesity." *Annals of the New York Academy of Sciences* 499, 55–65, 1987.

Welle, S. "Metabolic Responses to a Meal During Rest and Low Intensity Exercise." *American Journal of Clinical Nutrition* 40, 990–94, 1984.

Index